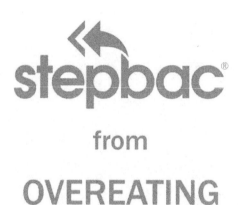

from

OVEREATING

Stepbac® Series - Book 2

How to stop eating too much using a New, Simple
method with Step-by-step Explanations and
Illustrations

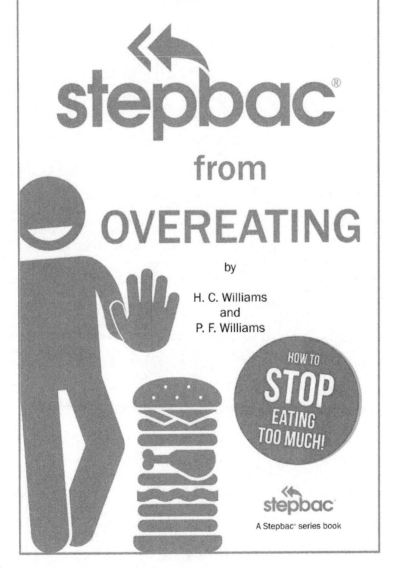

stepbac®

from

OVEREATING

by

H. C. Williams
and
P. F. Williams

HOW TO
STOP
EATING
TOO MUCH!

stepbac

A Stepbac® series book

Copyright © 2018 H. C. Williams and P. F. Williams

Disclaimer:

This 'Stepbac® from Overeating' self-help book and the Stepbac® method provide advice, motivation and instructions for a simple physical action that can assist you in making a desired change in a specific area of your lifestyle.

Your results will depend on your own efforts, commitment and understanding of the method and any achieved results will vary from person to person. Stepbac® cannot guarantee that everyone will achieve their desired result or predict how long a change in lifestyle might last.

This book has not been written by health practitioners or doctors and is not intended or implied to be a substitute for professional medical advice from your doctor or other physicians, nor is it intended to be for medical diagnosis or treatment. This is not a medical handbook and the biological explanations in the book are greatly simplified interpretations created by the authors solely for this book. You should always consult a doctor regarding any concerns about your mental or physical health, and any symptoms that may require diagnosis or medical attention.

Stepbac® shall not be liable for any physical, psychological, emotional, financial, or commercial damages, including, but not limited to, special, incidental, consequential or other damages incurred, or alleged to have incurred, directly or indirectly, by the information contained in this book. If you are not ready to make a change in your lifestyle – or do not want to make any changes in your lifestyle do not read this book. If you feel any kind of physical or mental discomfort from trying to change your lifestyle during or after reading this book, please seek professional medical advice.

This disclaimer is prepared under and shall be governed by Spanish law.

SBS2 SFO AM-Ed1 V5.1-300320

Dedication:

Dedicated to Philip & Stacia with love.

Table of Contents

INTRODUCTION

This book is about four
things that make you want
to overeat - and one thing
to help you stop
overeating

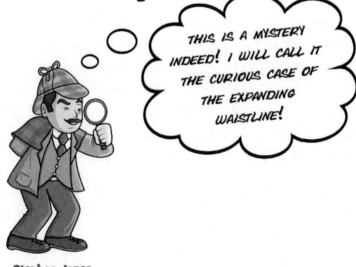

Stepbac Jones

Introduction

Introduction to Stepbac® from Overeating

"Stepbac® from Overeating" is the second in the series of "Stepbac®" self-help books. We have written "Stepbac® from Overeating" as an easy-reader book and we hope it will be fun, fast, interesting to read and easy to understand. We also hope it will be the most important book you ever read and that it will change the way you look at your eating habits and weight control.

What makes the Stepbac® method different? Everyone knows that eating too much is unhealthy, but very few people know how to effectively change their eating habits. Stepbac® is different because this book shows you how to change. "Stepbac® from Overeating" teaches you a very effective, practical and simple way to take back control of your eating habits and weight.

Many people in modern developed societies experience some weight gain from their mid-thirties or even mid-twenties. Modern life has made us more sedentary and by the time we reach our midlife many people have gained quite a significant amount of weight. By then we are busy and maybe a bit lazy, and we struggle to find the time and energy to shed the pounds and get back to our younger and natural weight. The waistline just seems to keep expanding and the weight seems harder and harder to control.

If that has happened to you, or is happening to you, then we think that the Stepbac® method described in this book can help you. We know how you feel, because both authors of this book went through the same weight gain; in our thirties and forties we put on weight, and for a few years it felt impossible to lose it again.

But then things changed. We started to take what we called a "Stepbac® from Overeating" - and it worked! We used our Stepbac® action as a tool to change all our bad overeating habits and to kill food cravings, and that enabled us to control our weight. Using Stepbac® we gradually dropped down to our natural and healthy body weight - the one we were at in our mid-twenties and it stayed there! Using the Stepbac® method also meant our health improved, our energy levels went up and our happiness levels soared. In fact we liked the Stepbac® method so much that we wrote this book about it.

The "Stepbac® from Overeating" method is neither a short-term weight loss diet nor an exercise system. Stepbac® is a simple way for you to understand why you have lost control of your weight and a simple way for you to take back control of the food that you eat so that your body's natural hunger process can control your natural weight. Another way we like to put it is that Stepbac® is a way for you to stop letting the food industry use your body as its trash can!

"Stepbac® from Overeating" teaches you, by using simple, step-by-step explanations with over 40 easy-to-understand diagrams, exactly how you're being tricked into feeling hungry when you're not actually hungry; how you're being tricked into eating too much - what we call overeating; how you're being tricked into eating low-grade food full of sugar - what we call fake Candyfood; and how you're being tricked into buying too much food - what we call overshopping.

The method is explained completely in this book. There are no extra treatments or additional products to buy. It's all in this book and it's all 100% natural.

"Stepbac® from Overeating" teaches you how to Stepbac® to the time when you were at a healthy natural weight and helps you to stay there. Stepbac® teaches you to change your unnatural overeating habits and by doing so take back control of your weight. When you have finished reading "Stepbac® from Overeating" you will know how to defend yourself against Candyfood and take a Stepbac® to a natural hunger cycle and natural eating and food shopping habits, which will enable you to take a Stepbac® to a healthy, natural body weight, so that your life can be better, happier, healthier and longer.

It's not possible to Stepbac® in time to become a younger person in years, but you can Stepbac® in time and go back to your younger health and weight. That will make you feel younger, because you will be healthier, feel better and have the same kind of energy and joy that you had in your youth.

When you have finished reading this book, we hope you will know how to start losing your extra weight and how to take the first of many Stepbac® actions to help you regain your natural weight and energy.

We are confident that "Stepbac® from Overeating" can help you understand why you're gradually becoming more and more overweight - and how you can stop weight gain and reverse it into weight loss, like we did.

How can Stepbac® help you control and lose weight if it is not a diet method? What most people generally term as "dieting" is to lose a few pounds in a few weeks, which, in our opinion, is a waste of time and money. We think it's the wrong approach to healthy weight control. Think about this. Hundreds of diet methods and diet foods have been available since the 1960s, so why is the news still full of stories about the rise in the number of overweight and obese people in almost every country in the world? Some of our own family members have been dieting all their lives - and yet they never seem to lose weight.

How can Stepbac® help you if it is not an exercise method? Well, fitness videos and gyms have been around since the 1970s. Same thing. Waistlines have expanded since the 1970s, so gyms don't seem to help most people. Of course some moderate daily exercise is essential for good health, but the evidence seems to suggest that for most people diets and fitness centers don't help them lose weight. So what does work?

"Stepbac® from Overeating" works. It teaches you a simple method - that anyone can learn - to change your eating habits so that you eat less food and eat less often. The best way - and really the only long-term way - to lose weight and to stay at your natural healthy weight, is to learn how to change your eating habits, change your attitude to modern food and change your lifestyle.

"Stepbac® from Overeating" will show you how people living in the developed Western world have been tricked into learning unnatural eating habits - or, more accurately, unnatural overeating habits. Most people eat too much and too often. They overeat. Even people who eat healthy food often eat too much of it. It is unnatural to overeat and our many overeating habits are what make us overweight. Our body is not designed to eat all day. Until recent times, most of us did not have unnatural overeating habits.

We think that the biggest reason that we eat too much is that the food industry adds massive amounts of sugar to food. The added sugar in almost all our meals and soft drinks hijacks our natural hunger process and tricks us into eating too much. The sugar in the food tricks our brains and makes us want to eat more often and, what is worse, it makes us eat when we are actually not hungry. We explain this in the Sugar chapter of this book.

"Stepbac® from Overeating" helps you understand how you're being tricked by sugar and by the food industry, and it teaches you how to "untrick" yourself from both using the Stepbac® method. When you understand how you're being tricked, then you can take a "Stepbac® from Overeating."

"Stepbac® from Overeating" can help you change all your overeating habits into one natural eating habit. Having one natural eating habit means that you will only eat when you're hungry and you will only eat the amount of food that your body needs to power itself and that your body is designed for. Eating naturally will mean that you stay at your natural weight and that your energy is at the right level.

This book is not about being thin or fat or about looks or fashion. It's only about how to take back control of your natural weight. In "Stepbac® from Overeating" we use the terms overeating and overweight. This is what we mean when we use those words (figure 1):

Overeat = is when we eat too much and we eat too often

Overweight = is what we become when we overeat.

Figure 1

To Overeat
is when we eat too much
and we eat too often

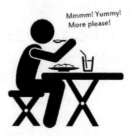

To be Overweight
is what we become
when we overeat

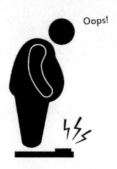

We prefer to use the word "overeat" rather than using the phrase "eat too much" because overeating covers both eating too often and eating too much and it has a clear connection with the word overweight. Overeating is not a word one hears very much. We often hear people saying the word overweight but not the word "overeat." Why is that? When people are overweight, they often talk about the need to exercise more. They rarely talk about eating less. We think most people don't want to eat less and they don't know how to eat less. So they pin their hopes on exercise. But most of us don't have time or energy to put in the necessary hours at the gym. Don't worry if you're the same. Daily movement is essential, but the primary reason many of us are overweight is because we overeat. So we will use the word "overeat" in this book.

In our opinion there are four main things that make us overeat. In this book "Stepbac® from Overeating" we will explain very clearly and with diagrams and illustrations what these four things are. We will show you how your body and mind have been attacked and hijacked by the food industry. Then we will teach you one thing to help you stop overeating. This one thing is a small and simple lifestyle change that can help you change all your unnatural overeating habits into natural eating habits, so that in future you will only eat the natural amount that your body needs to stay at your natural weight.

Don't worry. You don't need to plan a "chocolate funeral" or a "farewell to tiramisu party." You can still eat delicious food and, on occasion, have a treat, but after learning to take a Stepbac® you will only eat what you want to - and only when you want to. You will have total control. You will easily be able to control portion size and you will snack much less using Stepbac®. When you understand how you were tricked, you simply won't feel like eating all the time and you will not be manipulated by food cravings.

Before we start to explain how sugar tricks you into eating when you're not hungry and how you can Stepbac® and learn to control your eating and weight, let's first have a quick look at when and why the world started to gain so much weight. This is so you can understand that it was not always this way and that it does not have to be this way at all. What happened to us? How did the world go from slim to overweight in just 50 short years or 2 generations?

The way we were - what happened to us?

Why are so many people overweight in the 21st century? If we go back just 2 generations or around 50 years it is pretty obvious that hardly anyone was overweight at that time. Don't you find that strange? If we go back 75 years, which is about 3 generations we find that almost everyone was slim. Have a look at old photos of your great-grandparents and their generation, and you will see that most people were slender.

It's even stranger when one considers that they didn't have fitness centers or diets or free aerobics on the Internet or any advice from blogs, "YouTubers" and "influencers." No one had any of the information about the genetic structure of food or any of the health advice at our fingertips today. Most people, if they were lucky, had 1 cookbook and maybe an outdated 10-volume encyclopedia which was their "internet." No one had heard of calories, carbs, saturated fats or metabolism rates. But they were slim.

How could they know so little about healthy eating, not go to fitness centers, not be on diets, and not have exercise apps, pedometers and so on, and still be so slim? Or is the question really: how is it possible that we have all the tools and all the information that we need to stay slim - and yet many of us are overweight? How could this happen? It's a mystery. The mystery of the expanding waistline. Well, in this book we will do some detective work and lay the facts before you with a culprit and a solution. To help us along the way we would like to introduce you to our old friend and detective, Stepbac Jones, who will help us solve "The Curious Case of the Expanding Waistline!"

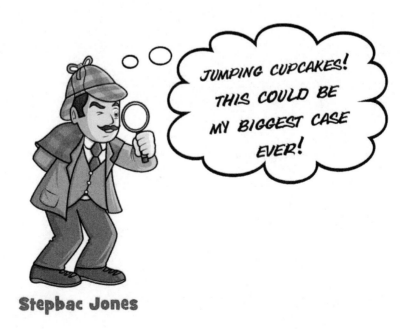

Stepbac Jones

We already know who the culprits are. You don't have to be Stepbac Jones to work that one out. The culprits are the food industry. What happened to us started in the 1950s when the food industry started messing with our natural hunger process and with our natural eating and food shopping habits. The food industry found out that they could hijack our bodies and our brains to fool us into overeating and overshopping - and we started becoming overweight (figure 2).

Figure 2

What happened to us?

Mr and Mrs Then in 1950s.
No diets, no fitness centers

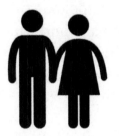
natural
slim weight

Mr and Mrs Now in 2010s.
Many diets, many fitness centers

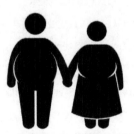
unnatural
overweight

Until the last decades of the 20th century, most people in economically developed countries were generally slim. They spent most of their lives at their natural weight. This was because people ate much less than we eat now. For some periods in history, tragic events such as famines and war naturally meant that there was less food available to eat, but in general people in previous centuries ate less because they followed more natural eating habits which were created by their bodies' natural hunger cycle.

People only ate at fixed mealtimes and that was because mealtimes were really the only times when food was available. Unless you cooked some food there were no snacks between meals and there were no "ready-made" dinners or takeouts. It was mostly women who cooked at home. Most men could not cook and were rarely in the kitchen.

Back then the homemakers, usually female, would prepare the family meals, which were eaten at fixed mealtimes. Portions were much smaller and meals were more natural and made from fresh ingredients in a balanced mix. Quite a few of the weekly meals were leftovers. There was less food at mealtimes and even the plates were smaller in size. In those days people got much more daily movement from walking, cycling and daily chores. So 2 and 3 generations ago people ate less and moved more, and this kept them slim. But that's not the whole story. The single most important reason that our great-grandparents were generally slim is that the modern food industry and food marketing industry did not exist. In today's world, food is often a finished product that is available 24 hours a day wherever we are. We eat more because there is more food. We eat more because food is everywhere. We eat more because we are constantly bombarded with marketing aimed at getting us to eat more and to eat more often.

Since the 1950s food production and distribution has become a massive industry. We use the term "food industry" in this book. By that we mean everyone associated with making and selling food which includes food manufacturers, food retailers, restaurants, food distributors and food marketers. Almost everyone in the mass food industry plays a part in redefining our relationship with food. Food used to be something that we only had to eat a little of each day to survive. Now food has become something that we crave, we glorify, we worship, we love and we live for! And that we are beginning to die for!

Since the 1950s the food industry has messed with our food, messed with our brains and tricked us into learning unnatural habits of overeating and overshopping for food. Have you seen that classic horror movie "Invasion of the Body Snatchers"? Welcome to the real-life version - starring you! By the time you have finished this book you will realize that your body has been "snatched" by the food industry.

That's an explosive statement, so let's explain what we mean in a little more detail. We humans are part of nature. We are part of the natural world. We are animals of a type called mammals. We have a natural weight that allows our bodies to work so that we can live a natural life using our bodies and all their parts. Now, we need some fuel to give us energy to power these bodies of ours so that they can work properly. The fuel that gives us energy is called food. We get the energy to power our bodies from food and drink. We need the right amount of food and drink every single day - not too much, not too little - but just about the right amount. If we get the right amount of food and drink, then we will stay at our "natural weight" and our bodies will work best. That is the way we human animals are designed. Our bodies function best at a natural weight. If our bodies get too much fuel we become overweight and our bodies don't work as well. If we get too little energy we become underweight and our bodies don't work very well. It's that simple. So we are designed to only need to eat the quantity of food that we need for energy. No less. No more.

This simple model for how a human body works best and how to power it best with food worked very well all the way from prehistoric times right until the 1950s. It worked well for our great-grandparents - people who were born around 1900. Then what happened? Well, in the second half of the 20th century - just 2 generations ago - everything about our eating and shopping habits started to change. Human eating habits suddenly started to change more in a few decades than they had in the previous 100,000 years or longer. Our bodies were snatched! Not by aliens, but by "alien" food!

Around the 1950s the modern food industry - and the food marketing industry - grew enormously. It started tinkering with our food and with our minds. We started the transformation from being people with a natural body weight and with natural eating habits to becoming unnaturally overweight people eating unnatural amounts of unnatural food. The result of decades of food tinkering is where we are now. We eat too much and too often. And we don't eat good food. We don't eat natural food.

The processed food that the food industry has tricked us into overeating is no longer natural food. The natural food that our great-grandparents ate at regular mealtimes every day powered their body with new energy. The unnatural food that we snack on and overeat many times a day, is stuffed with sugar, salt, sweeteners, chemicals and other "fake-food" ingredients. In the book we call this so-called modern food, "Candyfood". It's so full of sugar it's like candy for adults. It depowers us instead of powering us. In other words, Candyfood and "fake-food" steal energy from our bodies instead of giving us energy. It's not natural food and it's not real food. It's Candyfood! We don't think supermarkets should be called food stores any longer. They are candy stores for adults.

Most of the food in supermarkets today is highly processed and manufactured to taste amazing! It is actually incredible how amazing most food tastes nowadays. The problem is that natural food simply does not taste that amazing and should not taste amazing. Natural food is basically fuel and energy for our body so that we can stay healthy. Nothing more. Most natural food tastes good but not mouthwateringly amazing. Candyfood tastes amazing but no one can live off candy and stay healthy. So, sorry folks, Candyfood is unnatural and it's killing us!

People hardly ever eat natural food any longer. Our great-grandparents did it all the time but we almost only eat Candyfood! We eat boxed-up, plastic-wrapped, factory-made processed fake food that is full of sugar and additives. It tastes so good, it's almost better than candy, and because it tastes so great, we eat too much. We overeat. We hardly ever eat natural size portions any longer. We overeat every time we eat. And even after eating bigger portions at every meal, we still snack between meals. After all the overeating we often feel full, bloated, tired, ill and lethargic because we're overweight, and yet we still keep eating; we can't stop, we crave more food. Just like candy. Kids don't stop eating candy until they feel sick and even then they can keep eating till they are sick! That's how we adults eat food now. We don't stop till we drop (figure 3).

If you saw what a portion of natural food actually looks like, you might be surprised - it's actually a very small portion. A natural portion almost looks tiny by modern standards. It might be 1 small piece of meat or fish, a few potatoes or rice, and some vegetables. You would also probably be surprised at how little food we actually need to keep our weight natural and stay healthy.

Figure 3

Food to Candyfood

Mr and Mrs Then ate natural food

Before the 1950s we ate at regular mealtimes and we ate smaller portions of natural food that provided the right amount of nutrition to power our bodies and keep us at our natural weight

Mr and Mrs Then

Mr and Mrs Now eat Candyfood

In the 21st century we eat more often at irregular times, and much larger portions of unnatural Candyfood that is low on nutrition and makes us overweight

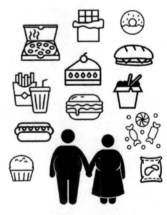

Mr and Mrs Now

We think it's safe to say that many people are now addicted to Candyfood, mostly because of the added sugar. We have become Candyfood junkies. Instead of being healthy energetic humans with a natural weight, natural food habits and natural energy from eating natural food, we shuffle around all day, moaning about our ill-health and lack of energy, searching for our next hit of Candyfood. We have become Food Zombies (figure 4).

Figure 4

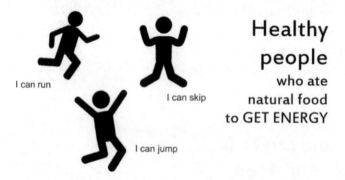

Food Zombies

How we were

I can run

I can skip

I can jump

Healthy people who ate natural food to GET ENERGY

How we are now

Food Zombies shuffling around all day looking for the next sugary snack of unnatural food that STEALS OUR ENERGY

"hungry!"

"sugaarrgh"

"must eat!"

We are Food Zombies! The food industry tricks us into craving Candyfood all day. It tricks us into overshopping, overeating and becoming overweight. Candyfood steals our energy instead of topping it up. It's as if the food industry has implanted a chip in our brains - only it's a potato chip! Modern humans constantly buy and gobble up massive amounts of low-quality Candyfood that the human body does not need. Our bodies pack it on as fat instead of burning it for energy. The food industry has invaded our bodies - they have taken control of our bodies. They make massive amounts of money off the misery of being overweight. The only defense that the food industry can offer is that no one forces you to eat too much. But when you reach the end of this book, you might feel, as we do, that being tricked into overeating is not very different from being forced into overeating.

"Stepbac® from Overeating" shows you why your body wants to overeat and how you can change a lifestyle of unnatural overeating into a lifestyle of natural eating by using the Stepbac® method. When you know how to Stepbac® then you can take back control of what you eat and thereby control your weight.

We are surrounded by food all the time.

Before the arrival of processed food, refrigerators, fast-food franchises, takeouts and so on, most people only ate at mealtimes at home, at work or, occasionally, in restaurants. Food was not available between meals. Even in the home, food was mostly made with fresh ingredients. Nowadays more people live in suburbs and cities than in rural areas. In the cities we are surrounded by food all the time. Food is everywhere we go and we are constantly tempted by machines, ads, smells and sights to have a snack. Almost all of it is Candyfood. The bottom line (no pun intended) is that we eat too much, and more often than not we overeat, because we are surrounded by food 24/7 (figure 5).

Figure 5

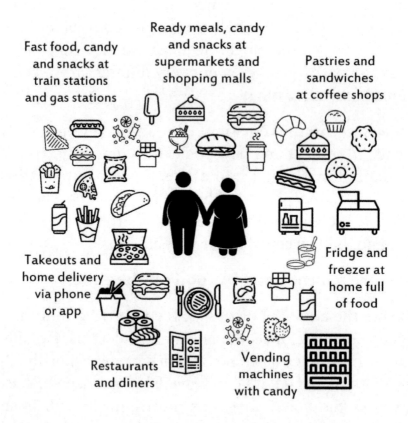

We are surrounded by food all the time

Fast food, candy and snacks at train stations and gas stations

Ready meals, candy and snacks at supermarkets and shopping malls

Pastries and sandwiches at coffee shops

Takeouts and home delivery via phone or app

Fridge and freezer at home full of food

Restaurants and diners

Vending machines with candy

Thanks for reading our introduction to "Stepbac® from Overeating", which we hope helped you to understand why controlling body weight has become such a problem for many of us. Now let's focus on solving the problem. In this book you will learn a simple way to take back control of your weight and to Stepbac® to a natural and healthy weight. Read on.

Chapter 1

OVERVIEW

Overview of the four things that make you want to overeat

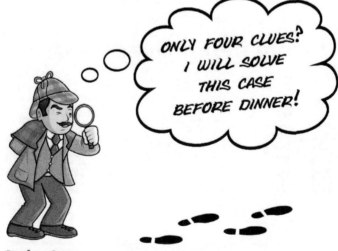

ONLY FOUR CLUES?
I WILL SOLVE
THIS CASE
BEFORE DINNER!

Stepbac Jones

Chapter 1 - Overview

Overview of "Stepbac® from Overeating"

The Stepbac® method is a combination of two things: Stepbac® information and a Stepbac® action. We chose the name Stepbac® because you will be taking a "step back" to a time in your life before you started to overeat and when you had a more natural weight (figure 6).

Figure 6

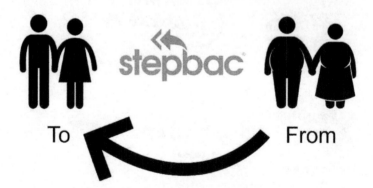

Stepbac®
from being Overweight

Generally speaking there are four main things in our modern lifestyle that make us want to overeat.

These four things are sugar, habits, cravings and food marketing.

The Stepbac® from Overeating method works as follows. First you read one chapter each about the four main things that make you want to overeat, which as we just mentioned are sugar, habits, cravings and food marketing. Together we call this the Stepbac® information. Then you read one chapter in which we teach you one thing to make you stop overeating, which we call the Stepbac® action.

When you have read the four chapters with the Stepbac® information and one chapter about the Stepbac® action, we hope you understand the Stepbac® method (figure 7), which will help you eat less and gradually step back to a natural weight, which will also mean a healthier lifestyle.

Here is a quick overview of each of the four things that make you want to overeat. Don't worry if you don't understand it all fully yet. This is only an introduction to the more detailed Stepbac® information about these four parts of overeating. We will go into detail about each one in the next four chapters.

Figure 7

The Stepbac® method

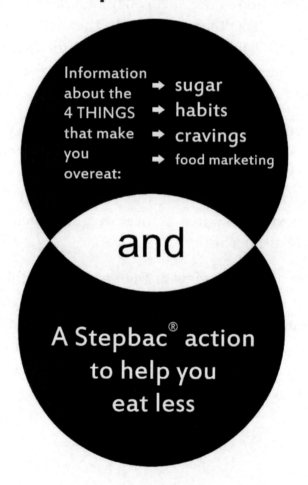

Information about the 4 THINGS that make you overeat:
→ sugar
→ habits
→ cravings
→ food marketing

and

A Stepbac® action to help you eat less

1. Sugar:

Sugar is the first of the four things that make you want to overeat. Sugar is the general name for sweet soluble carbohydrates. Sugar is not what we would normally classify as a drug, but it is commonly accepted that sugar affects our brain in the same way as addictive drugs do - and some scientists label it a "drug" for that reason. Sugar is highly addictive and can cause food addictions very similar to drug addictions. Sugar can also cause withdrawal symptoms and cravings, which lead us into a cycle of overeating. Basically sugar makes us want to eat too many sweet things and it makes us overeat. You will learn all about sugar in Chapter 2.

2. Habits:

The second of the four things that make you want to overeat is habit. In Chapter 3 we will tell you how your brain creates an overeating habit - actually many small overeating habits - that makes you eat more. Your overeating habit is created and powered by sugar and cravings.

3. Cravings:

The third of the four things that make you want to overeat are cravings. If you haven't eaten for a while, then your brain generates a craving to eat. This craving to eat is linked to your eating habits. We will tell you more about how this works in Chapter 4.

4. Food Marketing:

The last of the four things that make you want to overeat is food marketing. We are surrounded by food. We are tempted with food all day. Eating is portrayed as something blissful and associated with complete happiness. This is how food companies want to market eating to us, especially to young adults. Food marketing tempts us into overeating.

The Stepbac® method to stop overeating has been designed to help you understand and take control of these four things that make you want to overeat, using the Stepbac® information and the Stepbac® action (figure 8).

Figure 8

For the Stepbac® method to work you must

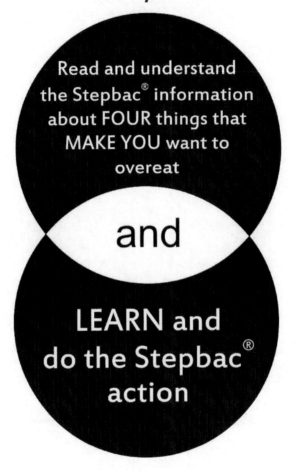

Read and understand the Stepbac® information about FOUR things that MAKE YOU want to overeat

and

LEARN and do the Stepbac® action

Chapter 2

SUGAR

The first of four things that make you want to overeat

I KNEW IT! IT'S MY OLD ENEMY SUGAR! THIS TIME I AM READY FOR YOU!

Stepbac Jones

Chapter 2 – Sugar

Figure 9

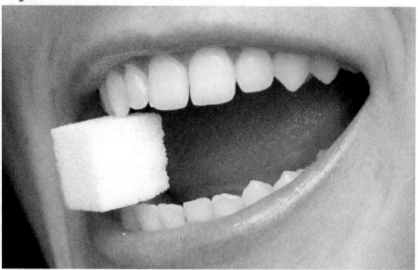

Sugar is the single biggest cause of overeating (figure 9). Unnecessary sugar is added to a lot of our food. There are some other things which are added to processed food that make us overeat, which include items like salt and fat, but the sugar in food is the single biggest reason that we overeat. Much of our food and many soft drinks have way much too much sugar in them. We are not talking about the sugar that you add to your tea or coffee or sprinkle on desserts. We are talking about sugar that the food industry pours into nearly all the processed food that we buy in the supermarket.

Now most of us would probably agree that food tastes much better with sugar or sweeteners. Remember the Pepsi challenge advertisements? People were asked to choose the best tasting cola in a blind taste challenge between Pepsi and Coke. Participants almost always chose Pepsi; apparently even the top manager of Coca Cola once chose Pepsi in the challenge. The reason Pepsi always won the challenge was that at first sip Pepsi tasted sweeter than Coke because of its higher sugar content. Sugar does taste very good. Most people would agree that sugary food tastes better than natural, healthy food like potatoes, vegetables etc. Most of us often have cravings for something sweet but very few have a craving for a carrot, a potato or a turnip.

Many of us know that delicious food tempts us to overeat which then makes us overweight. We all know that choosing not to eat sugary food and sugary drinks would be much healthier. We even know that sugar has very little nutritional value. And finally many of us tend to feel that if we could choose to be slim, then most of us would rather be slim than overweight because we know that being overweight does bring some discomfort, some unhappiness and can lead to bad health. If we know all that, then why do we keep overeating and struggle with being overweight? Why not just eat less? Why do we like sugar so much? And why can something that nice be so bad for us?

Few people know much about the science of sugar – why it is so addictive and what actually happens inside our brains when we eat sugar. We just know that sugar is sweet and that we love it. Here's a fun fact. Did you know that our brains actually encourage us to eat sugar? Amazing, but true. Our brain wants us to eat sweet things - it even gives us a reward by making us feel happier after eating something sweet. Doesn't that seem odd? Why would our brain want us to eat sweet things when we are told over and over that too much sugar is bad for us? The answer to that question is in your mouth and in your brain. Time to have a closer look at what sugar is and how it affects us.

What is sugar and what does it do to us?

What is sugar? Sugar is a carbohydrate that is found naturally in the sugar cane plant. There are other sources of sugar and there are other kinds of sugar, but the one we modern humans know best is white table sugar, which is made from sugar cane syrup. Some sweet tasting food has natural sugars in it, like fruit, but most of our processed food has ordinary sugar added to it in order to make it taste better - and to make us overeat. Without sugar, salt and fat, most processed food would either be tasteless or even taste bad and we would eat less of it.

In a moment we will show you what sugar does to your brain but first a couple of lines about the history of sugar so you understand how the sugar industry evolved. Until fairly recent times sugar was a luxury item that only the very rich could afford. Modern methods to refine sugar were not invented until the early 19th century, and before that sugar was very expensive and not available for mass consumption. Before sugar became available to everyone, the sweetener that most people used for cooking was honey, if they could afford it.

From the 1950s the amount of sugar in food and soft drinks exploded. Why? Because the food industry added sugar to almost everything we eat to make it taste better, to make it last longer and, most importantly, to make us eat more.

The added sugar started messing with our brains and disturbing our natural eating process. We became addicted to sugar. Some experts will say that sugar is not a drug, so it cannot be addictive. Is that true? If you go online you will find that many "experts" argue about the definitions of food and of drugs. Who cares, though? Does it matter if sugar technically is a food or is a drug, or both? What matters is that sugar is being added in unnatural amounts to most of the food we eat including many daily food items like bread, cereals, yogurt, soft drinks and, of course, snack bars and candy. What matters is that sugar has an addictive effect and creates strong cravings which attack our brain and hijack our natural eating process and reset it on a new course: to make us overeat. Wow. Sugar is a health terrorist. How can something sweet be such a terrible force?

Here come some answers. Fasten your seatbelts. This chapter about sugar is a bit of a bumpy ride with technical bits and can seem a little bit boring to read, but we have tried to make it as easy and light to understand as possible so please try and get through it. If you know your enemy, then you can defeat it. Sugar is your enemy. You need this information about sugar to be able to find out how you're being tricked by sugar into overeating and to kill your sugar cravings and stop overeating.

What happens in our body when we eat?

We humans are the species called "homo sapiens" (which is Latin for "wise man"). Our body, including our brain, was created hundreds of thousands of years ago and has slowly evolved since then. In many ways our bodies and brains have not changed over all that time. We function in the same way as prehistoric humans did. We need energy to function and to survive. We get this energy from eating food. The prehistoric human body and brain was equipped with a hunger cycle and an eating process to help us eat and survive. We still have that.

This natural eating process is what made early humans feel hungry, so that they would eat when their energy level was low. In addition to hunger feelings their body encouraged them to eat by giving them a reward for eating. The reward was a feeling of pleasure. This happy feeling came from a chemical called dopamine which was released in the brain after eating. The function of dopamine was to make people feel good and to make them eat again the next time they were hungry. Hundreds of thousands of years later modern humans like us still have the very same natural eating and hunger instinct as our prehistoric ancestors.

This eating process that we have in common with our prehistoric forefathers is controlled by our brains. It has two main parts. The first is the taste buds on our tongue and the second is what we call the "hunger survival cycle". Let's start with our taste buds. We have the same taste buds as prehistoric humans. Taste buds were made to help us make the right choices about what was safe to eat (figure 10).

What are taste buds?

We all have between 8,000 and 10,000 taste buds spread across the surface of our tongue. They are the tiny bumps that you can see on your tongue. The function of our taste buds is to send messages to the brain about how something tastes. A taste could be something sweet, sour, bitter, or salty - or umami. Those are the five basic tastes. Don't worry if you haven't heard of umami; it's quite a new word that describes the taste of something that is neither sweet nor sour, salty or bitter - like meat or soup or cheese (figure 10).

Figure 10

Taste buds

All taste sensations come from all regions of the tongue, but different parts are more sensitive to certain tastes

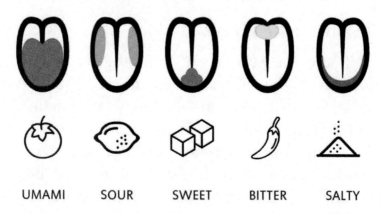

UMAMI   SOUR   SWEET   BITTER   SALTY

Our taste buds today are exactly the same as the ones that the earliest humans of our species had on their tongues. In prehistoric times humans survived entirely by instinct and their taste buds were much more important to them, because their taste buds instinctively helped them to decide what was good and, more importantly, what was safe to eat, which was crucial to their survival. Taste buds provide this help by reacting in certain ways when we put something in our mouths. Taste buds register immediately whether food is sweet, salty, sour or bitter. The taste buds of modern humans have the same function.

Bitter food can be poisonous. Our taste buds identify a bitter taste and signal our brains to spit it out because it could kill us. The taste buds which are positioned at the very back of your mouth are the ones that are most sensitive to bitter tastes. They are the taste buds that will try to prevent you from swallowing something when it reaches the back of your mouth because it is very bitter and perhaps deadly.

Taste buds can also identify a sweet taste. When our taste buds identify sweet tasting food, a signal is sent to our brains with the message that this is safe to eat. And that's not all; for eating sweet tasting things we get an extra reward from our brain – an extra shot of dopamine to make us feel happy (figure 11).

Figure 11

Prehistoric humans

| SWEET TASTE | BITTER TASTE |

Sweet things
are GOOD to eat
for energy and
brain rewards
with a feeling
of pleasure

Bitter things
are BAD to eat
because they could
be poisonous and
brain does not
reward with
feeling of pleasure

The reason for this happiness reward of dopamine is simple. Our prehistoric ancestors had very different food sources and very different eating habits compared to ours. Food was not conveniently stacked on shelves in a shop. It had to be grown, found or hunted. This was very hard work and our prehistoric ancestors did not always get their hands on much food. They ate mostly for survival and not for pleasure, unlike us. We mostly eat for pleasure.

Early humans did not have candy and sweets. The few natural sweet foods that early humans ate were mostly berries and fruit. Berries and fruit contained high amounts of energy, which was crucial for survival. Generally speaking, the more energy there was in food, the less you would need to eat to survive, although you would still need a varied diet. Because sweet foods were only available in limited amounts and for a limited season, the pleasure centers of the brain were activated by sweet tastes. That is why humans feel so very happy when they eat sweet things. This happiness reaction to sweet food was originally intended to make sure that early humans ate as much sweet food as possible to get the high energy boost, whenever it was available.

This dopamine "bonus" happiness reward for eating sweet things when you could was a brilliant brain process for the early humans who lived hundreds of thousands of years ago. Sweet food was a rare thing and a good thing to eat. To put it another way, for prehistoric humans sugar was a friend and a good friend at that.

Sugar was our friend

So sugar was our friend and you don't build a defense system to keep friends out. On the contrary, you welcome friends inside. Eating too much sugar and becoming overweight was not a problem in prehistoric times, so prehistoric human brains simply did not have a defense system or barrier to stop anyone from eating too much sugar. Early humans had taste buds to warn them away from bitter poisonous foods but sugar was a friend so sugar got the welcome mat. Now we are hundreds of thousands of years and generations later in the 21st century and we modern humans still do not have a defense system against sugar. Sugar has now become our enemy, but we are defenseless against it. And that is what the food companies found out.

Sugar is now our enemy

Sugar has now become our enemy number 1, because in modern times instead of being scarce, sugar is abundant. There is way too much sugar in almost everything we eat. We eat Candyfood and have become Food Zombies because of sugar cravings. Why is there so much sugar in all our food? The answer is that the modern food industry pours sugar into food. They found out in their laboratories that in the 21st century the human brain still does not have a defense system against sugar. They know that our brain puts out the welcome mat for sugar. That is why they are putting extra sugar in food, to make us overeat (figure 12).

Figure 12

From friend to enemy

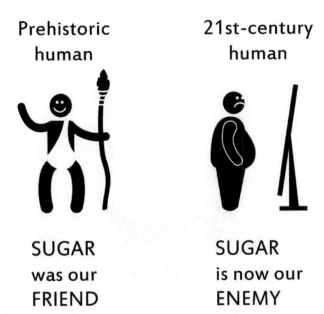

Prehistoric human	21st-century human
SUGAR	SUGAR
was our	is now our
FRIEND	ENEMY

The more sugar in food, the more we overeat

The food industry knows that when it puts more sugar in food, we eat more. We overeat. When we overeat, we buy more food. When we buy more food, the big food companies make more money. We become overweight. The food industry doesn't care if we become fat and unhealthy. It doesn't care because its bank accounts become very fat and very healthy (figure 13).

Figure 13

Food industry is filling us with sugar

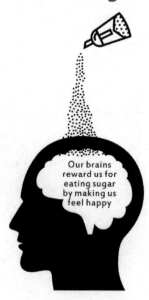

Our brains reward us for eating sugar by making us feel happy

Our brain has no defense against sugar. We are rewarded with feelings of pleasure for eating and drinking sugary food and drinks

It's that simple. The unnaturally large amounts of sugar in modern food make us overeat. As we explained in the introduction, the modern food we eat is very sweet and that's why we call it Candyfood. We eat much too much Candyfood instead of natural food - and we drink much too much Candywater instead of water. This means that most people have a sugar addiction. It doesn't matter if your particular guilty pleasure is chocolate, muffins, cupcakes, cookies or something else. The cravings and the pleasure are caused by the sugar content.

A sugar addiction "hijacks" our brain's natural ability to monitor our natural food needs. Sugar changes and perverts our natural eating habits by creating fake feelings of hunger. The fake hunger feelings caused by sugar trick us and make us eat when we are not actually hungry. And that, to use a not very scientific term, sucks!

Let's take a closer look at how the brain is supposed to manage our body and our daily food needs, and at how we are now all being tricked by sugar into overeating.

How is our brain being tricked?

Our brains were developed way back in prehistoric times but they are still pretty smart. In many ways they are much more sophisticated and advanced than modern computers and smartphones. However, unlike a smartphone or a computer, our brains were not developed last year by an engineer in an IT company in Silicon Valley or assembled in a factory in China a month ago. Our brains were created and developed hundreds of thousands of years ago by nature.

Smartphones and computers get upgrades and new models are released every year. Our brains do not get upgraded. Smartphones and computers have new apps and firewalls to protect them from malicious virus attacks. Our brains do not get new, updated defenses.

This means that, although our brains are still considered to be the fastest and smartest computer processors on the planet, a human brain can very easily be tricked by things in the modern world. For example, our brains have no upgrade or firewall app to defend us against sugar. Our brains can't protect us from sugar. We don't have a "sugarwall" (figure 14).

Figure 14

Sugar is hijacking our brain

Smartphone
made
in 2000s

Human brain
made hundreds of
thousands of
years ago

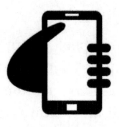

Last upgrade
thousands
of years ago!

Smartphones and
computers are
updated and upgraded
all the time. They can
be protected from
malicious attacks

Our human brain
computer doesn't get
upgrades and has no
protection from
malicious tricks like
sugar addiction

A computer virus goes into a computer system and corrupts it into doing things that we don't want it to do. Sugar is almost like a virus. It infects our brain, corrupts it and makes us do things we don't really want to do. How sugar does that is by creating cravings that infect and corrupt our natural hunger cycle and that create fake feelings of hunger. The fake hunger feelings make us do something most of us really don't want to do, which is to eat when we're not hungry. Doesn't that sound a bit like a virus?

To understand how sugar does this damage, let's look at how our brain manages our natural hunger and eating processes.

How our brain and eating process work

The human brain dates back to the beginning of human evolution. The brain is the control system of the human body - you could say it is the body's computer. Its basic function is to monitor and control our bodies to keep us alive and well. In our brains we have some fundamental and prehistoric survival instincts embedded. They are there to help us survive. No one has to learn these human survival cycles - they are already pre-programmed in our brain and they are active from birth, from the very first breath we take. When a baby cries it is often one of the natural survival cycles making it cry to tell someone that it's hungry, thirsty, cold or tired.

Human survival cycles

Human survival processes are very complex, so we have created a simplified interpretation for the Stepbac® books, which we call human survival cycles (figure 15).

Figure 15

Human Survival Cycles

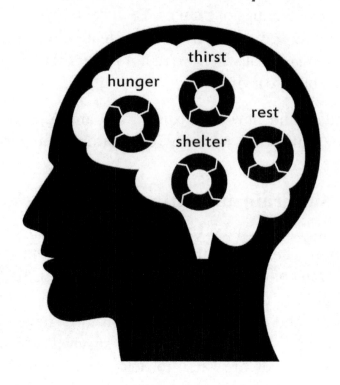

The four most important natural human survival cycles are hunger, thirst, rest and shelter. These are the ones that we can, to a certain extent, control ourselves, prioritize and even temporarily postpone. These four human survival cycles are so important to staying alive that they are essentially the brain's top priority.

One of the most important natural survival cycles is the hunger cycle. The human body runs on food, and food is our energy source. Food is what fuels us and gives us energy to function. Our bodies' hunger survival cycle can be compared to the way a car only functions when we keep it fueled. Without fuel a car cannot drive, so we have to monitor the fuel level. A car has a fuel gauge with an empty and a full mark. When the fuel is low and near the empty mark, a warning signal flashes to tell the driver to put some fuel in the car before it stops.

The human hunger survival cycle works in a similar way. Many people think that the feeling of hunger comes from actually having an empty space in your stomach. That is not how hunger works. It just feels that way. Look at the diagram (figure 16).

Figure 16

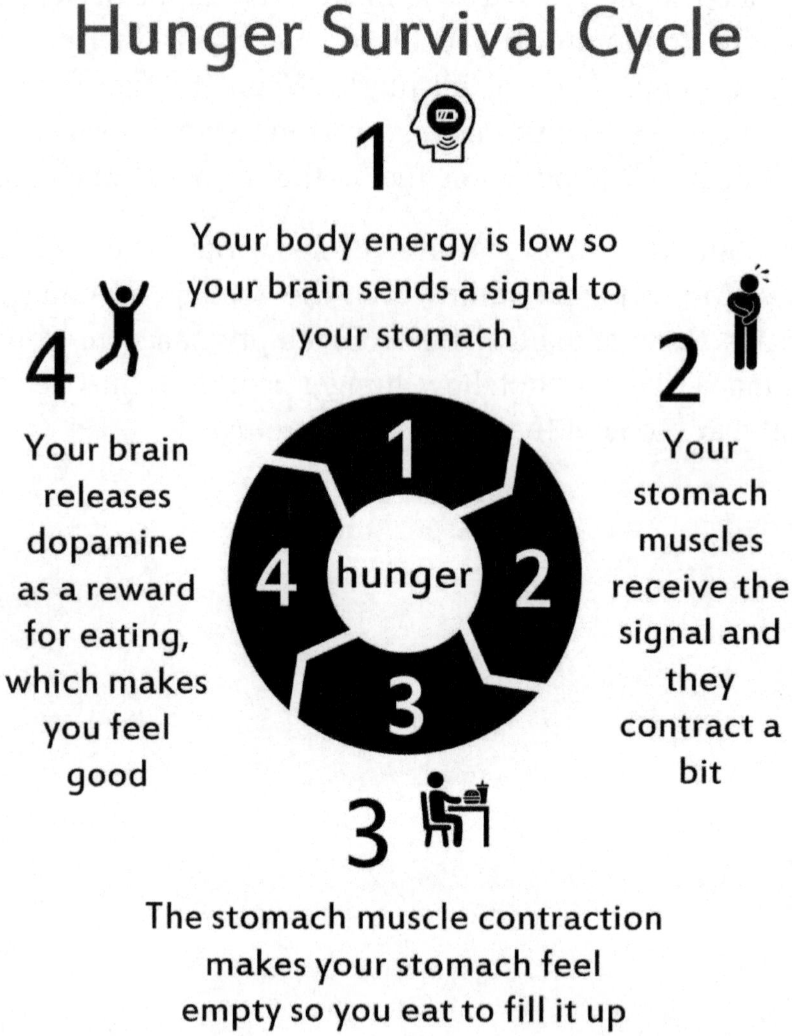

Hunger Survival Cycle

1

Your body energy is low so
your brain sends a signal to
your stomach

4

Your brain
releases
dopamine
as a reward
for eating,
which makes
you feel
good

2

Your
stomach
muscles
receive the
signal and
they
contract a
bit

3

The stomach muscle contraction
makes your stomach feel
empty so you eat to fill it up

What happens is that your brain is constantly monitoring the level of your body's energy levels, a bit like a car's fuel gauge. Our energy comes from food. When our energy level is low and near the empty mark, the brain makes us eat. The brain does this by releasing hormones that send a signal to your stomach muscles telling them to contract and shrink, so that you will feel hungry and will eat (number 1 in diagram above.)

The stomach gets the message and contracts a little, which means it shrinks slightly (number 2 in the diagram), and this stomach contraction is what makes you think you have an empty stomach. In your mind you might have an image of an empty space. You might also feel a bit drowsy and low on energy when you're hungry - this drowsiness and lack of energy is also a reaction caused by signals from your brain that is telling you to refuel by eating food to renew your energy levels.

So you eat some food (number 3 in the above diagram) because you feel hungry and need to top up your energy levels. Then what happens? When you eat, your brain stops sending "eat now" signals and your brain rewards you for obeying the signals! Your brain rewards you with a shot of dopamine (number 4 in the diagram). The dopamine reward makes you feel happy. Dopamine is a natural drug in our brain. It is a neurotransmitter that produces feelings of happiness; in simple terms, dopamine is the brain's feel-good reward drug. Each time you get a warm, happy, comfortable feeling, it happens because dopamine was released by your brain. It is also released when you do something nice for someone else, or when you do something that you really enjoy.

Dopamine plays a very important role in the body's survival cycles because, as you can see in the diagram, it is the reward that we get from our brain during the survival cycles. Every time you do something that is good for you, like eating, your brain rewards you with dopamine to make sure that you enjoyed eating and to encourage you to do it again.

This is how the hunger survival cycle works. Remember this is a very simplified visual interpretation created by the Stepbac® authors to help explain these complex processes. In the same way, this simplified visualization of how our brain works can be used to explain some of the other ways your brain monitors and controls your body.

By using similar human survival cycles, your brain can control many different functions in your body. Your brain can tell you to drink when you're thirsty, to sleep when you're tired and to stay warm when you're cold. These actions are all controlled by similar human survival cycles. And the wonderful sensations that come from climbing into bed when you're really tired or having a cold drink when you're really thirsty are the dopamine rewards from your brain for completing the sleep survival cycle and the thirst survival cycle.

Sugar hijacks your hunger survival cycle

We are explaining all this to you so that you can understand how the added sugar in your food manipulates and corrupts your natural brain cycles. And why it is happening. The human body does not need sugar in food to survive. Sugar has no essential nutrients. A varied diet of meat, fish, vegetables and fruit provides all the nourishment (and some natural sugars) that a human needs. If you never ate a lump of sugar again, you would not suffer and you would not die from a lack of sugar. Your health would actually improve. You would live a longer and healthier life than most people who eat too much sugary food and drink.

Sugar is a big ingredient in food products today, but it was not in our diet until quite recently. Since the 1950s the food industry has poured extra sugar into our food, drinks and snacks, and created the industry of what we call Candyfood.

The vast amounts of sugar in our food make us become addicted to sugar. The feeling of pleasure every time you eat something sweet creates a sugar addiction. A sugar addiction works exactly in the same way as a drug addiction. You feel better when you eat sugar than when you don't eat it.

Like any other addiction, when you're not eating sugar, you start to build up a craving for sugar. These cravings trick our brain. We think we are hungry, but actually we are not. What we're feeling is a sugar craving. The sugar craving infects and hijacks our normal and natural hunger and eating cycle, and it tricks us into feeling hungry by starting a "fake" hunger cycle. Sugar has become a hunger terrorist (figure 17).

Figure 17

Sugar Survival Cycle
tricks you into feeling hungry

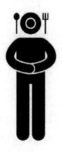

REAL HUNGER
feelings are your
body's way of
telling you
it needs energy

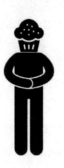

FAKE HUNGER
feelings are
just sugar CRAVINGS to
make you eat when
you're not hungry

That is essentially why we overeat. Your natural hunger survival cycle has been hijacked by sugar. The sugar craving makes you think you're hungry when you're not hungry. The sugar cravings "fake-start" the hunger cycle. By hijacking your hunger cycle, the craving forces your brain to signal your stomach to eat something even though you're not actually hungry. You're being tricked by sugar into eating when you're not hungry (figure 18).

Figure 18

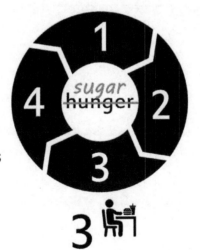

HIJACKED
Hunger Survival Cycle
sugar

1

You're not hungry, but you get a craving for SUGAR which forces your brain to signal your stomach

4

Your brain releases dopamine as a reward for eating which makes you feel good

2

Your stomach muscles receive the signal and they contract a bit

3

The stomach muscle contraction makes your stomach feel empty, so you eat to fill it up

You're not actually hungry. You only think you're hungry. You think you need to eat food. What you're actually feeling is a craving for sugar. Remember that you only need to eat for energy to survive. You only need a specific and quite small amount of food a day to power a healthy body at a natural weight. But the sneaky sugar cravings are tricking you into eating when you don't need to eat for energy. If you don't need to top up your energy then you're being tricked into overeating. You will eat more often if sugar cravings constantly "hijack" your natural hunger cycle and supersize it with "fake hunger" feelings. It spirals out of control and the supersize hunger cycle now dominates your life, making you overeat all the time.

Let's have a look at how your brain looks with your hijacked and supersized hunger survival cycle (figure 19).

Figure 19

Hijacked Hunger Survival Cycle

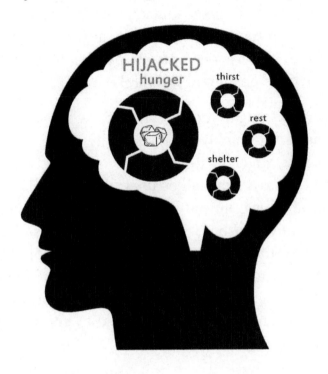

Wow! Look at the size of brain's hunger survival cycle after being supersized by fake hunger from sugar. This supersize hunger survival cycle is bigger and more powerful than all the other natural survival cycles like thirst and the need for shelter and rest. The hijacked hunger cycle has become the dominant survival cycle because, for most people, it now feels like you're hungry and thinking about food all the time. Food has become the most important thing in your life! You can't stop eating because each sugar craving "fake-starts" the supersized hunger cycle and creates fake hunger feelings many times a day. Instead of only eating the natural food you need when you're genuinely hungry, you eat too much, snack more often and buy too much food so you can have snacks within reach all day. You're not hungry but you eat anyway. You crave Candyfood! You've been taken by the food industry. You have become a Food Zombie!

That's what sugar does. This is why we become overweight so quickly and so easily. This is why so many of us struggle to just stay overweight and not become obese. Sugar makes us want to eat all the time. We humans have no natural defense against sugar, so we must now learn to make one. We must learn to reject this Candyfood -gobbling, Food Zombie lifestyle and get back to eating a natural amount of food each day to reach and stay at a natural weight and keep us powered at a natural level. We need to get back to the way nature designed us.

Think of it like this. Car manufacturers build a car with a certain size engine to power the car based on a certain type of fuel. What would happen if you overloaded the car and filled it with the wrong fuel? It wouldn't work very well or for long. Our bodies are like a machine. We can't fill it with the wrong fuel - or overload it - and then expect our engine (the heart) to keep working normally. When our bodies become overloaded with weight the human skeleton can't support the extra weight which leads to joint problems and the heart can't pump blood around the body, leading to heart problems and strokes. The "fat" bottom line is that we break down. Just like an overloaded vehicle with low grade gas would eventually do.

So how much should we eat and what should we eat? Good question. However, as we said at the beginning, this is not a diet book so we don't provide specific eating suggestions and we only teach you to eat much less. We want you to understand how little food we actually need to eat every day to stay alive and to stay healthy. It's hardly anything. Men only need 2,200 calories a day and women only need 2,000 calories. You might think that you would be hungry the whole time if you ate that little. You would be wrong. Sugar cravings trick you into fake feelings of hunger, but if you stayed away from sugar, you would not feel hungry all the time even if you ate only 2,200 or 2,000 calories a day (figure 20).

Figure 20

How many calories a day do we need to be healthy?

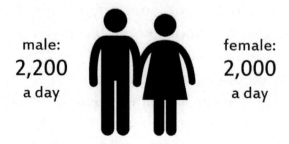

male:
2,200
a day

female:
2,000
a day

**If we eat this amount of healthy food
every day we will not feel hungry often**

We need to eat very little a day to avoid feeling hungry. Try searching online for pictures of what 2000 calories of healthy food actually looks like. You might be surprised. It's not much. Or search for pictures of the number of calories in popular fast food meals and drinks. It's a lot. Many of us eat all our daily calories in a single meal. Then we eat two more meals in the same day. And have snacks in between meals!

Ask yourself this: if we overeat all the time then why do we so often feel hungry? Why are we ready to eat all the time? Why are we constantly talking and thinking about food and our next meal? Are we really hungry? NO. Are we fake hungry with withdrawal symptoms from Candyfood sugar cravings? YES. If you really felt hungry and had genuine hunger pangs, then you would probably want some real food. But do we crave an apple, a banana, a turnip or a potato? No. We crave a burger, a sandwich, a muffin, a candy bar or a donut.

Are you beginning to understand now? That you're not actually hungry. That you just crave sugar – you're "fake hungry." It's a pretty sneaky trick, isn't it? Add extra sugar to food and snacks. People are addicted to sugar. The sugar cravings from the addiction hijack our hunger cycle and trick us into eating more and buying more.

How much and what should we eat?

First of all we should eat less. In Chapter 6 we will teach you how to do that. We will teach you how to take a Stepbac® from Overeating. What should we eat? We should eat more natural food and less sugary food. There is plenty of natural food around and it is quite cheap compared to the packaged food we are surrounded by every day. That's the good news. The bad news is that natural food is not very sweet and not always very tasty. What we modern humans in the developed world seem to have forgotten is that natural food, which is safe to eat for humans, can almost be described as tasteless or bland. Natural food does have taste. Nowadays some people call the natural food taste "Umami." Umami is the "fifth taste" to follow salty, sweet, sour and bitter. Umami is a savory but bland and neutral taste.

Examples of rather taste-neutral food are potatoes, rice, cauliflower, turnips, cabbage, nuts, apples, pears, and even meat and fish. These bland tasting foods are safe to eat, natural and healthy. But who wants to eat only potatoes, or only rice, or only cabbage? Well there are ways to make bland food taste a little better without sugar and we will talk a little more about this in the final chapter, but the important thing to understand is that we have to make food less important in our lives. We have to stop glorifying food. We have to be less greedy. We can still be "foodies" but we can't be "Candyfoodies." We must eat for energy, not for pleasure. We should eat for sustenance, not for joy. If we want to reach and stay at our natural weight we should take a "Stepbac® from Overeating" and start eating natural food in sensible amounts.

If we eat natural food and only the amount needed to power our body then we will always stay at a natural and healthy weight. Why is this important, you might ask? It's important because we humans are not designed to carry a lot of extra weight. Our heart can't support it. Our skeletal frame can't support it. Our organs can't support it. It's simply not a feature of the human body. There is no sticker on our bodies when we are born that says, "This body can support three times its natural weight and still function!" Being overweight is possible for a while but it's not healthy and it's not a good option for long-term health and happiness (figure 21).

Figure 21

The human body is not designed to be overweight

Think of your body like a car. A car that has to transport you on your journey of life from the beginning to end. The engine of your body is your heart. The fuel is your food. The car frame is your skeleton.

A car is designed with an engine, which runs on fuel to power the weight of the car frame with a normal load.

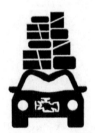

Would a car drive as well and at the same speed if you put bad fuel in it every day and overloaded it a little more every day? It would drive worse and worse and eventually break down.

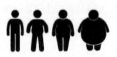

Your body will work worse and worse and eventually break down before the end of your life journey if you are powering it with bad food and overloading it a little more every day.

Conclusion Sugar chapter

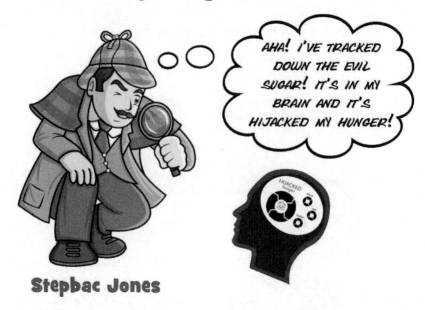

Stepbac Jones

What did Stepbac Jones find out about sugar? He found out that sugar is a very powerful substance, that some scientists even call a drug. Excessive amounts of sugar have been added by the food industry to most of the food that we eat. Why? To make us eat more. The food companies know that if they tried to sell natural food without sugar and in healthy amounts, then they would not make much money. First of all, natural food is not as tasty as sugary food. And second, if we all only ate the 2,000-2,200 calories a day that we actually need to be healthy and survive, then we would not eat very much at all. So there is little profit in people eating only natural food in healthy amounts.

Stepbac Jones found out that the lure of greater profit made the food industry add a lot of sugar to our food.

We modern humans eat far more sugar that our prehistoric ancestors did and even than our grandparents did. Stepbac Jones also found out that the reason sugar makes us overeat is because sugar messes with our natural hunger process. Sugar does this by hijacking our natural hunger cycle and "fakestarting" it to make us feel hungry when we are not actually hungry.

Fake hunger signals trick us into eating. Eating when your body does not need food or energy is overeating and will make you overweight. The sugar creates an addiction and cravings that force us to eat more than we should. Most people would love to eat less but they can't - because of the sugar addiction.The bottom line is that we have become overeating, overweight Food Zombies addicted to Candyfood.

That was Chapter 2 about sugar. Well done for getting through it. In Chapter 3 we tell you about the second of the four things that make us overeat: habits. We look closer at how the food industry and our sugar addiction take advantage of our natural daily eating habits to create unnatural overeating habits.

Chapter 3

HABITS

The second of four things that make you want to overeat

THE SECOND CLUE IN THIS CALORIFIC CASE IS HABITS! WHERE ARE YOU MY SWEETIES? STEPBAC JONES WILL FIND YOU!

Stepbac Jones

Chapter 3 - Habits

Welcome back. Now we're going to give you the Stepbac® information about habits and how they work, specifically our eating habits. Habits are the second of the four things that make you want to overeat, and bad eating habits make it very hard to stop overeating. Habits can become a very good friend of sugar and Candyfood. Habits can make you overeat without you noticing or thinking about it. Overeating is a habit, a bad habit.

You've doubtless heard of "bad eating habits" and heard messages about changing to "healthy eating habits." And we know that we want to "break the habit" or "kick the habit" when it comes to habits like having a snack with every coffee. We know it isn't easy, because we think that "old habits die hard!" Habits are "ingrained" inside us.

We might talk a lot about changing our habits without doing anything about it because we think it's easier to talk about it than actually kicking the habits. But in fact an old habit does not have to "die hard" at all. An old habit can actually "die easy" because it can be changed quite easily once you know how to change it. When you have finished this book you will know how. This book teaches you how to change your bad overeating habit into a natural eating habit.

But before we get to the actual Stepbac® method, we need to learn and understand more about habits. So now we're going to teach you all about habits, how they work and how they can be changed. Again, a word of warning. You might find this a bit dry and boring, but please hang in there and try to get through it. To change your overeating habit, it's very important that you understand how habits work in your brain. Once you know that, you will find it much easier to stop overeating using the Stepbac® action that we will teach you later in this book. Without this information the Stepbac® action will not work.

What are habits?

First let's look at habits in general. We asked a lot of people what they thought habits were. The most common answers were:

"Something we do without thinking about it"
"Things we do every day"
"Something we do automatically"

All the answers above are correct. Habits are behaviors and actions that we do automatically. We do them without conscious thought. We don't have to think about them. This is because habits are simply a copy or a repeat of a sequence of actions that we have done many times before.

How are habits formed?

Where do habits come from? All habits, good and bad, are acquired. We learn habits. We learn different habits at different times of our lives. Some habits are learned at a very young age. Walking is a habit. Cycling is a habit. Using a knife and fork is a habit. Brushing your teeth or looking both ways before crossing a road are typical habits. We all have many habits. As a child you learn how to do many things, so that later in life you can just do them automatically and without thinking. If we had to think about every footstep we take, we wouldn't get very far. We learn many habits as children, but we also learn many as adults. We can learn or acquire new habits throughout our lives. At any time in our lives, we can learn new good habits and we can learn new bad habits.

What is the difference between a good and a bad habit? In general terms a good habit is something that we want to do. It is something that we like doing or that gives us some satisfaction. We do it of our own free will, like doing the dishes straight after a meal, or folding clothes after taking them off. Those are examples of good habits, which we want to keep on doing. A bad habit, on the other hand, is something that you do against your free will. Normally we don't want to keep bad habits. We want to stop bad habits. A bad habit is something you don't really want to do, but you can't stop doing it. You can't help it. Nail biting is an example of a bad habit. There's no sugar or addictive substance in your nails, so why is it so difficult for some of us to stop biting our nails? Because it's a habit.

Examples of bad habits

Bad habits are the ones that you can't stop or control very well. Nail biting, smoking, snacking on chocolate, eating too much, drinking too much alcohol, taking drugs, checking your Facebook page for updates every 5 minutes - things like that. These are all habits that you've learned - or were tricked into learning. Some bad habits don't have an addictive substance and some do; smoking has nicotine, drinking has alcohol, drugs have chemicals, food and snacks have sugar.

Examples of good habits

Good habits are the automatic actions that you like doing and don't want to stop doing. We all have many good habits. Some of them we acquired at a very young age, like walking or using a knife and fork. Some we learned as older children, such as brushing our teeth or cycling. And there are some good habits we learn as adults, like shaving in the morning and washing the dishes right after a meal. There are many good habits.

What are not habits? To help you understand what habits are, let's also have a few examples of things that are not habits. Things that we don't do every day and we can stop doing whenever we want are not habits, but interests. Going to the movies, playing Monopoly and going to the beach - those are not habits. They are not automatic actions that we do without thinking.

So now you know that habits are sequences of actions that we perform without thinking about them. They are automatic actions. Studies have shown that brain activity is very low when we perform a habit sequence. This is because the brain already knows what to do when it has learnt a habit sequence and so it doesn't have to think much about it. The brain has stored a sequence for each habit we do on a regular basis. For example, using a knife and fork to eat is a habit. We do the same thing every time we use a knife and fork to eat, so our brain doesn't spend any energy at all thinking what to do with these two metal objects. It just gets the knife and fork habit sequence from the habit storage room and starts it, so we can use a knife and fork without thinking about it. The brain is on autopilot.

When our brains have to think, there is brain activity and our brain uses energy. The thinking part of our brains - the wiggly-looking part - is called the cerebral cortex. In the middle of our brains and underneath the cerebral cortex, there is a smaller and more primitive area of brain tissue, which is called the basal ganglia. (Thanks brain scientists for the easy-to-remember names you give things!) The basal ganglia part of the brain is not used for thinking. Until recently no one really knew what the purpose was of the basal ganglia. But recent studies have revealed that the basal ganglia is where our brains store our habits (figure 22).

Figure 22

The Cerebral Cortex is the wiggly
outer part of our brain that we use for
active thinking

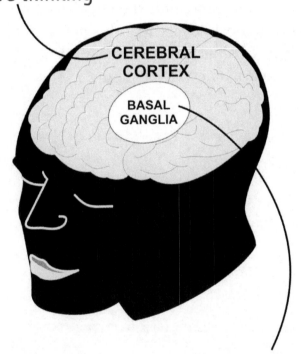

The Basal Ganglia is a smaller inner
part of our brain where we store the
habits that we have already learned

Basically it works like this. As we've just seen, all habits
are acquired. In other words all habits are learned.
When we learn a habit sequence for the first time, there
is huge activity in our thinking brain part - the cerebral
cortex. It is working very hard. The first time you
picked up a knife and fork, your cerebral cortex was

bursting with activity to try and understand and learn what to do with these metal things. Which way up do I hold them? How do I use them together? And so on. It feels very easy for us now to use a knife and fork to eat, but look at a child learning to eat with a knife and fork. It takes a long time, and the child's brain activity and concentration while learning this new habit sequence is very high. Look at the next diagram of what happens while we learn a new habit (figure 23).

Figure 23

While learning a habit

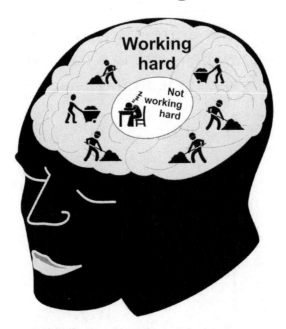

While we are learning a habit the wiggly outer part of our brain (cerebral cortex) is working hard, but the inner, habit-storage part of the brain (basal ganglia) is not working hard

As the child learns how to use a knife and fork, and gets better and better at it, the sequence becomes more and more familiar, and the child thinks less and less about it. After a while, eating with a knife and fork becomes an automatic habit sequence. Something the child can do without thinking about it. It becomes a habit (figure 24).

Figure 24

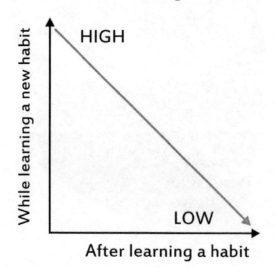

Cerebral Cortex activity level is high while learning a habit and low after learning a habit

HIGH

LOW

While learning a new habit

After learning a habit

After using a knife and fork has become a habit, then the thinking activity in the cerebral cortex goes down to almost zero whenever you pick up a knife and fork. And which part of the brain does the work now? Yes, the basal ganglia. When you pick up a knife and fork now, the activity level in your basal ganglia goes up (figure 25).

Figure 25

After learning a habit

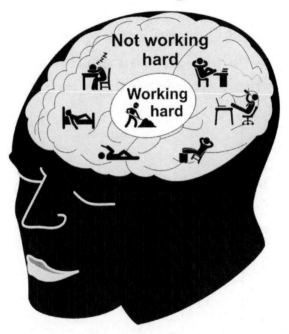

After we have learned a habit, the wiggly
outer part of the brain (cerebral cortex)
does not work hard anymore, but the
inner, habit-storage part of the brain
(basal ganglia) works hard to fetch the
habit we already have learned and stored

The first time we learn a habit sequence there is high
activity in the cerebral cortex outer part of the brain,
and low activity in the basal ganglia area of the brain.
After learning a habit sequence, there is low activity in
the cerebral cortex outer part of the brain, and high

activity in the basal ganglia area of the brain (figure 26).

Figure 26

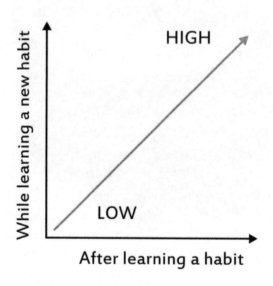

Basal Ganglia activity level is low while learning a habit and high after learning a habit

This brain process of storing and fetching habits is almost like installing and using apps on a smartphone. When we learn a new habit sequence it's a bit like installing a new app on our phone. But most apps on a phone are only loaded when we use them. Until we use them many apps just reside in the phone's storage. In the same way, a habit is a pre-programmed sequence stored in your brain. A habit sequence is only loaded by the brain when we need it. For example, the teeth brushing habit sequence is a habit stored in the basal ganglia. We only need the sequence of actions to brush our teeth twice a day. When we need it, the brain fetches it, and we use it automatically without using any brain effort to think about it.

Another example is driving. After you've learnt how to drive, you don't need to think much about things like changing gears, pressing brake pedals or letting in the clutch. You don't have to think about how to put the engine into reverse gear. You've done all that so many times that the brain has all those actions stored as habit sequences. When you drive, each habit sequence is fetched and each action is automatic and without conscious thought. The first time you took a driving lesson your wiggly cerebral cortex part of the brain was probably at 99% activity. Your entire brain was concentrating on remembering everything, getting the timing right and trying not to hit anything. By the time you passed your driving test, your brain had learned all these actions and they had become habits stored in the basal ganglia. When you drive now your brain loads your driving habits like an autopilot system.

Why does the brain make habits?

This method of learning habit sequences, storing them and loading them when we need to use them happens because the brain needs to reduce effort, where it can, to be efficient. The brain has limited processing power and energy, which is a bit like a smartphone too, so storing habits means that the brain can free up thinking and processing power for other things. When you drive this means the brain can be more efficient and can be used for thinking processes like scanning the road, evaluating possible danger ahead and making quick decisions. Your brain would probably not be able to cope very well with complex traffic situations if it hadn't already stored the habitual driving sequences for all the basic actions of driving, such as changing gears and pressing pedals.

What activates a habit?

We have now learned that the level of brain thinking activity is low after we have learned and stored a habit sequence. We don't have to think about a habit - it is in our basal ganglia with all our other habits. Like an app on a phone, a habit is there when we need it. But how does the brain know when to load a particular habit sequence? Do we have to tell the brain when to load and run each habit routine (figure 27)?

Figure 27

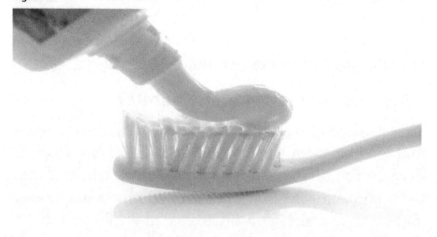

"Good morning brain. I really need the teeth brushing habit sequence now. I'm in the bathroom and late for work already. Hello! Wake up brain. What do I do with this stick with hairs on? And what's this plastic tube thing? Please activate the teeth brushing habit sequence." Well, it's not quite like that, but almost. You don't have to pester your brain to help you find your stored habit sequences; instead it works like this - the brain is always looking for a sign to tell it if you need any of the habit sequences it has stored. We call this sign a trigger. A trigger is something the brain detects that tells it we need to use a particular habit sequence.

For example, if the brain sees a toothbrush or detects the smell of toothpaste, then it activates the teeth brushing habit sequence. The teeth brushing habit sequence was triggered by the toothbrush; the brain recognized the toothbrush and got the toothbrush habit sequence ready. Let's look at the habit sequence in a bit more detail. The brain is always on the lookout for a trigger, so that it can load a habit sequence from the basal ganglia.

A habit sequence has three parts:

a TRIGGER > an ACTION > a REWARD (figure 28)

Figure 28

Habit sequence

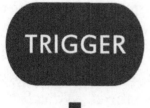

TRIGGER. A habit sequence begins with a trigger. When the brain spots a trigger, it loads the habit routine that it has stored

ACTION. The action in a habit sequence is done automatically without conscious thought

REWARD. The reward for completing a habit sequence is when our brain releases dopamine, which is the drug the brain can release to make us feel happy

Let's see some examples of how this process works with good and bad habits. This is our habit sequence for brushing teeth (figure 29):

Figure 29

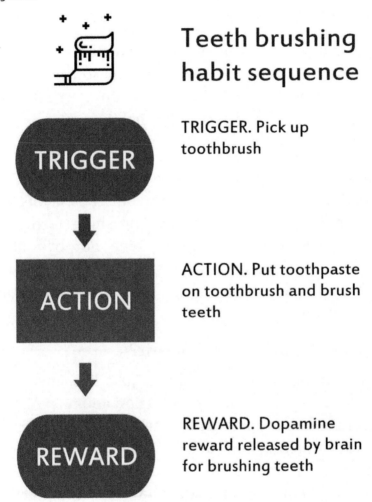

Teeth brushing habit sequence

TRIGGER. Pick up toothbrush

ACTION. Put toothpaste on toothbrush and brush teeth

REWARD. Dopamine reward released by brain for brushing teeth

When you've brushed your teeth, part of the habit sequence for teeth brushing is that we run our tongue over our clean smooth teeth and sense the clean minty taste. This gives us a feeling of satisfaction that is a tiny feeling of happiness and well-being. This little feeling of well-being comes from the dopamine released by your brain as a reward for doing the teeth brushing action and completing the teeth brushing habit sequence.

Not all habit sequences end with a dopamine reward, but many habits do. We take the time to learn habits that end with a dopamine reward because we enjoy the satisfaction of completing the habit sequence and getting the dopamine reward.

So now we know how a habit sequence is formed and where it is stored. We want to keep our good habits and our useful habit sequences like brushing teeth and driving, but we don't want to keep our bad habit sequences. Overeating is one of our worst habit sequences, so let's have a closer look at our overeating habit sequence now.

What is the overeating habit?

An overeating habit sequence is just like any other habit sequence. It has a trigger, action and reward. The overeating habit starts with a trigger that makes us want to take action and eat something, and it ends with a dopamine reward from the brain. There are many overeating habit triggers. After an overeating habit is activated, we automatically respond with the action of eating.

What triggers an overeating habit?

Have you ever thought or said something rueful like "Well, I'm not really hungry but..." or "I shouldn't really be eating this..." or "One teeny-tiny piece can't hurt..."? Our mother used to say, "It won't make you fat till tomorrow!"

Thoughts and words like that often pop up when you're offered something to eat, or see food in a shop or café. That is because just seeing a tasty snack is a trigger. Seeing someone else eating is a trigger. Smelling food is a trigger.

You might have a feeling that you're not really hungry and that you probably shouldn't eat whatever it is you're being offered, but you just can't help yourself. The trigger makes you reach out automatically to take one and eat it, even as you tell yourself that you really shouldn't (figure 30).

Figure 30

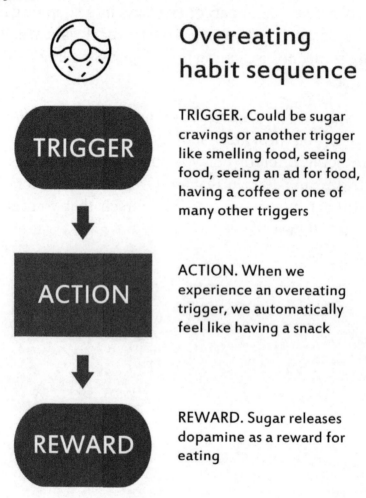

Overeating habit sequence

TRIGGER. Could be sugar cravings or another trigger like smelling food, seeing food, seeing an ad for food, having a coffee or one of many other triggers

ACTION. When we experience an overeating trigger, we automatically feel like having a snack

REWARD. Sugar releases dopamine as a reward for eating

This is a good example of how you overeat out of habit when exposed to an overeating habit trigger. Often you might not even have time to think or say any rueful words before the food or snack is in your mouth. That is because putting something in your mouth is an automatic habit. You're on autopilot.

You may think you snack and overeat because you love food, but the truth is that most of the time you're being manipulated and controlled by your overeating habit triggers. In reality you're hardly conscious of the fact that you're snacking too much, and you seldom pause to think whether you're actually hungry or whether something is healthy or not.

Sugar cravings are the strongest overeating triggers and can mentally distract you so much that you can hardly think of anything else until you have put something sweet in your mouth. We will look at this trigger in more detail in the cravings chapter.

There are many other daily overeating habit triggers. Drinking a cup of coffee can be an overeating habit trigger - who drinks coffee these days without a snack? The smell of freshly baked bread. Advertising signs with special offers for food and drink. Online and TV ads. Seeing people eating on TV or in movies. Seeing other people eating. These are all eating habit triggers and they are everywhere. For example, aromas from a restaurant or food smells in a mall, where food smells are deliberately blown down the aisles to blast shoppers coming towards cafés. Try eating something tasty outdoors and take note of how many people look at your food with envy in their eyes, thinking "where did you get that? Why is that person eating and I'm not? I want one! I could kill you and take your snack!" These overeating habit triggers are all around us all day.

Like any other habit sequence, there are three parts to an overeating habit sequence. The first part is the trigger that makes you want to eat. The next part is the action, which is putting something in your mouth. Finally the overeating habit sequence ends with the reward, which is dopamine to make you feel good. We get dopamine just for eating and we get extra dopamine from the sugar in Candyfood, snacks and sweets. As we told you in the sugar chapter, sweet tastes trigger the brain into releasing an extra dopamine reward for eating something tasty/sweet.

Our in-house detective Stepbac Jones discovered that we actually have many overeating habits, not just one. We often speak about overeating being "a bad habit," as if overeating is just one habit. But people who overeat actually have many different overeating habit sequences. Each overeating habit sequence is a bit different, because it has a different trigger. This is why it can feel hard to eat less and lose weight without help, because you have to kick many overeating habits, not just one.

The next diagram illustrates many of the overeating habit sequences (but not all of them!) Each overeating habit sequence has a different overeating habit trigger, and each trigger leads you to the automatic action of eating something. As you can see from the diagram, a person who overeats has many overeating habit sequences stored in their basal ganglia, not just one (figure 31).

Figure 31

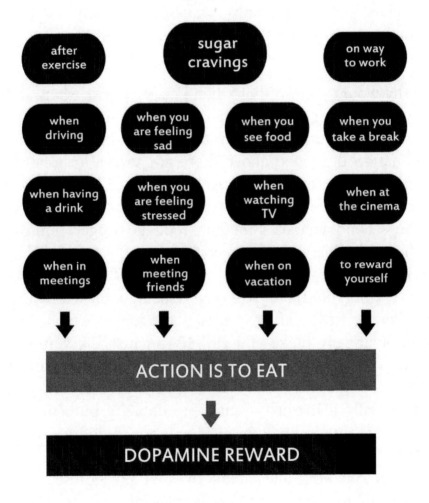

Overeating habit triggers

Look at the overeating triggers in the previous diagram - you can see that sugar cravings are one of the strongest overeating habit triggers. But there are many other overeating habits. Even after a meal, when we're not really hungry and don't have sugar cravings, we might still feel the urge to eat something.

Here's an example: Imagine that you have just eaten a meal in a restaurant and are meeting someone for a drink. You're not hungry, but when they order some nachos with their drinks, you eat some too and that might even prompt you to order something else to nibble on.

Why would you do that when you have just eaten and your body doesn't need energy? You do it out of habit. Or to be more precise, out of many habits. In the situation described above there are several overeating habits which are automatically triggered to make you eat. Seeing food is the first trigger. Seeing people eat is the second trigger. Smelling food is trigger number three. Having a drink or coffee could be trigger four. Having your friends offer you food and tempt you a little could be trigger five. You're being attacked by five different overeating habit triggers, which all automatically make you eat! If you just ask yourself, "am I hungry?", the answer would be "no, you've just eaten." But it's likely that you will eat anyway. Especially if it's just a snack, a nibble, a bite. In this kind of situation willpower is outgunned and loses the fight. Willpower might help against one trigger. That's one on one - but one against five! Willpower loses. And there might be more habit triggers later in the day. A late-night snack on the way home from a gas station. Some snacks you have in the car. A snack from the fridge when you get home. All these are habits taught to you by the food industry to keep you eating which we'll explore in detail in Chapter 5. Willpower is defenseless against that many overeating triggers - unless it has some help from a method like Stepbac®.

Conclusion: Habits chapter

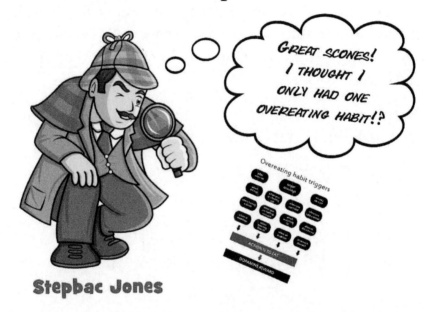

Stepbac Jones

Stepbac Jones has discovered that habits are things that we can do without thinking about them. They are automatic patterns of behavior called habit sequences that are learned and stored in the basal ganglia part of our brain. Habit sequences always have a trigger, an action and a reward. We do many things every day on autopilot by using our stored habit sequences, which are only activated when we need them, a bit like apps on a smartphone.

Stepbac Jones also made the important discovery that you have many overeating habit sequences and not just one overeating habit. There are many daily overeating and snacking triggers that trick you into automatically loading an overeating habit sequence, making you eat a little something even when you're not hungry.

Now you know all about habits and soon you'll be able to use the Stepbac® method to replace all your overeating habits into one new Stepbac® from Overeating habit. Yes. One new habit instead of all the old ones.

But first we need to look at the third of the four things that make you want to overeat: cravings.

Chapter 4

CRAVINGS

The third of four things that make you want to overeat

CUNNING CRAVINGS THEY MAY BE – BUT I WILL CATCH THEM – WAIT AND SEE!

Stepbac Jones

Chapter 4 - Cravings

What are cravings?

You have just learned that an overeating habit sequence consists of: a TRIGGER > an ACTION > a REWARD. And you learned that our many different overeating habits make us automatically reach out for something to eat without really thinking about it.

The added sugar in processed food, which we call Candyfood, also creates strong cravings that are closely linked to overeating habits. Sugar cravings can even create new overeating habits. Let's try and understand how cravings work and how they can help create some habits.

Have you ever had a craving for broccoli? Or a craving for cooked asparagus, or boiled fish and potatoes? When was the last time you had a craving for any type of home-made soup or vegetables as a snack? Probably never, right?

As we mentioned in the Sugar chapter, humans do not have cravings for natural food. Natural food is only fuel to power our bodies with essential energy so that our bodies function well and we can stay alive. We are designed only to eat natural food and only when we are hungry. We are designed so that when we're not hungry, we don't think about natural food or have cravings for natural food. Natural food is quite bland and boring and tasteless. One might say it simply does not taste good enough to trigger cravings.

Cravings for sugary food are entirely different. We have many of them. They are created by the very tasty but fake and unnatural processed food that we call Candyfood. This unnatural fake food is usually full of sugar, salt and fats, which create cravings for more food and make us overeat.

How do cravings work?

Explained very simply, a craving is when you start thinking about how nice it would be to have something or do something before you actually get it or do it. A craving is often created by the combination of a habit sequence that contains an addictive substance like sugar or alcohol or a drug like nicotine. Most of us have experienced cravings for Candyfood like fast food, ice cream and chocolate. Smokers have cravings to smoke because of smoking habits and nicotine (see the book "Stepbac® from Smoking," if you're a smoker), and alcoholics and drug addicts have cravings for alcohol and drugs.

Here's an example of how a craving works. If you start thinking about how nice it would be to eat some chocolate, then you're already starting to anticipate the pleasure you will feel when you actually eat the chocolate. In other words, you're anticipating the reward of pleasure that you will get, before you actually get it (figure 32).

Figure 32

Craving

You have a craving when you start
thinking about the reward before you
complete the action

This anticipation of the pleasure we will get from eating chocolate is called a craving for chocolate, and it can be so powerful that many of us will take the time to find a shop, café or machine where we can buy anything with chocolate in it, if we don't have chocolate on hand.

Let's try to explain cravings in a little more detail. Let's say you love chocolate-chip muffins (we hope we're not making you too hungry with these examples!) and someone says "let's meet at 3pm at the pastry shop for coffee and a chocolate-chip muffin." Your brain will "jump for joy" in anticipation of the pleasure that you'll feel when you bite into a chocolate-chip muffin later that day. In other words, your brain is already telling you how wonderful this experience is going to be at 3pm.

If you can't stop thinking all morning about the delicious muffin you're going to eat at 3pm, then your brain is craving the pleasure that you will get from eating that muffin later. If you can scarcely think about anything else for the rest of the morning except a chocolate-chip muffin, then the craving has become powerful and is becoming an obsession.

If you go to the pastry shop as planned and eat your chocolate-chip muffin then you'll get the real reward of pleasure from its delicious taste, which you've been looking forward to all day. But if for some reason you can't make it to the pastry shop and you don't get your chocolate-chip muffin, then you won't get the reward of pleasure that you've been anticipating and craving all day. If your craving is not fulfilled, then the brain reacts with feelings of irritation, depression and maybe even anger.

How are cravings linked to habits?

Here's an example of how cravings link to habits. Let's say you start buying chocolate every day because you can't stop thinking about chocolate in the morning. Your craving for chocolate is what creates a habit of buying and eating chocolate. This is an example of how a craving can create and sustain a daily habit. After just a week or two, a new craving for chocolate in the afternoon might have created a new habit in your daily life: buying a little piece of chocolate on your way home from work.

Today you have many different overeating habits - and many of them were either created by cravings or are still powered by cravings on a daily basis. Every time you experience an overeating habit sequence trigger, which happens many times a day, your brain will immediately look forward to and anticipate the relief, and what you feel as "pleasure," from the sugar in the food or snack.

In other words, you will often feel a craving for food or a snack after an overeating trigger. But if for some reason you're denied that food or snack - either because you're using your willpower to try to lose weight or the convenience store is closed or you ate the last snack you had at home earlier then the food/snack craving will build into feelings of irritation, annoyance, depression and even anger. Some people use a new word for being hungry and angry that is "hangry!" Most of us don't get "hangry" often, but we're sure you know the feeling of wanting a snack and not getting it and will agree that it can feel difficult to focus or relax when a craving to eat becomes more and more dominating.

As we explained in the Sugar chapter, sugar has infected your brain and hijacked your hunger survival cycle by fake-starting it so that you feel hungry. This means you're constantly looking forward to eating something tasty very soon. You're craving snacks without realizing that your hunger is now being controlled by your sugar cravings that have helped create overeating habits. If you cannot get hold of a snack or whatever food or treat you were looking forward to eating, you will feel pangs of "fake hunger" (figure 17). You will feel a bit miserable and depressed, and can even become short-tempered, irritable and "hangry."

These feelings are called "withdrawal symptoms." These are very similar feelings to those that are experienced by drug addicts and smokers when they have not taken their drug for just a little while. Sugar withdrawal symptoms from not getting a chocolate snack can feel just as bad as the withdrawal symptoms that a smoker experiences when he or she is not able to smoke. This is because they are basically the same type of physical cravings.

Your brain was expecting and anticipating a happy dopamine reward from eating something tasty and sweet – but did not get it. The "fake hunger" pangs you feel when you have a craving for chocolate are the same "fake hunger" pangs that a smoker feels when he or she cannot smoke. Your brain is sending the same message to your stomach muscles to contract, so you get the feeling that you're hungry even if you just ate. To get rid of these pangs, a smoker will light a cigarette and people who overeat will reach for something to eat, often unnatural food, a snack, dessert or piece of chocolate.

Cravings are the third of the four things that make it difficult to stop overeating. Even when you have learned to change and control your overeating habits using the Stepbac® action, which we will teach you later in this book, you will still be challenged by an occasional craving for chocolate or snacks in certain situations.

But don't worry. You will learn to use the Stepbac® action to combat overeating habit triggers and kill snack cravings.

You will still be able to enjoy an occasional dessert or ice-cream, snack or piece of chocolate in the future, but the Stepbac® method will help make sure you do not have any daily snacking and overeating habits, and stop you creating new ones.

Conclusion: Cravings chapter

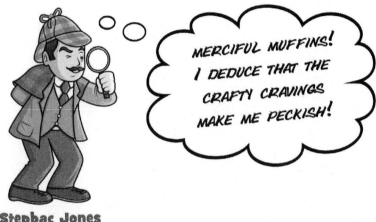

Stepbac Jones

In this chapter Stepbac Jones found out that a craving is when you start thinking about how nice it would be to do something before you actually do it. A sugar craving could be when the thought of a delicious-looking chocolate muffin makes your mouth water in anticipation of eating the cake soon.

Cravings often start when you see an overeating habit trigger, but have nothing to put in your mouth when you see the trigger. Your brain has already started anticipating the dopamine reward from the snack long before you actually get hold of the snack.

When you experience overeating or snacking cravings in the days after you start using the Stepbac® method, remember how they work. Cravings are easy to spot because you can feel them as "hunger" pangs and a feeling of mild sadness or irritation which can become worse. We will teach you how to easily deal with cravings in our Stepbac® action chapter. Now let's look at the fourth thing that makes you want to overeat, food marketing.

Chapter 5

FOOD MARKETING

The last of four things that make you want to overeat

GOTCHA! THE FINAL CLUE TO SOLVING THE CURIOUS CASE OF THE EXPANDING WAISTLINE!

Stepbac Jones

Chapter 5 – Food marketing

How we are being tricked by the food industry. In Chapter 2 we told you what sugar is, what it does to the brain and how the food industry adds unnecessary sugar to many kinds of food to try and make us eat when we are not hungry. We told you how most of the food that we now eat is not natural food, but what we call Candyfood. In Chapters 3 and 4 we learned about habits and cravings, and how sugar helps create habits and power the cravings that make us overeat. Sugar, habits and cravings are three of the four things that make us want to overeat. Now we come to chapter 5 and the last thing that makes us want to overeat: Food marketing.

Any good news in this chapter you might ask? Er... wait... erm... ah... well... there might erm.. let me check... nope! Sorry. There is a bit more bad news in Chapter 5. But there will be plenty of good news in Chapter 6, so hang in there. And our book will have a happy ending, we promise! But the bad news in this chapter is that you will find out that the food industry not only messes with our minds when we eat food. They also mess with our mind when we buy food! They have a super-sized bucket of sneaky marketing tricks to make us buy much more food than we need. Of course they don't call them sneaky tricks. They call them "persuasion methods."

Let's take a closer look at food marketing and advertising, food shopping and food distribution. You might be shocked at how much "persuasion" you're being exposed to.

Food advertising and marketing

Food advertising, marketing and branding is everywhere in modern life. We are surrounded 24/7. Food marketing is on TV, the Internet, billboards, websites, apps, in newspapers, magazines, radio, concerts, sponsorships and sports events. Unless you live in a mountain cave you can't avoid food marketing. Unlike some products, tobacco for example, food can be advertised almost anywhere to anyone, including children. There are very few limits on food advertising or what claims can be made in food adverts.

Before the 20th century, marketing almost didn't exist. There were no flyers in your mailbox, no loyalty cards, no special offers, no exotic food choices, no TV cooking channels and most households had one standard cookbook, often handed down from previous generations. Food was just fuel for the body, and anyway, there wasn't much of it around so there was little to advertise. Today everything has changed and we are surrounded by food marketing (figure 33).

Figure 33

We are surrounded by food marketing

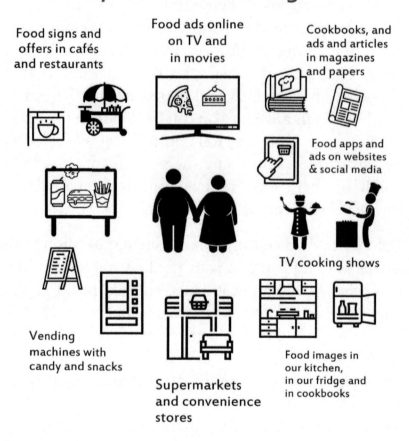

Food signs and offers in cafés and restaurants

Food ads online on TV and in movies

Cookbooks, and ads and articles in magazines and papers

Food apps and ads on websites & social media

TV cooking shows

Vending machines with candy and snacks

Supermarkets and convenience stores

Food images in our kitchen, in our fridge and in cookbooks

Food marketing generally focuses on one core message. The message is that eating makes you happy. Not just happy but the happiest you can be. The ultimate feeling of pure happiness. For that reason they want us to treat food like something to be glorified and almost worshipped. But ask yourself what the real purpose of food is? Is it A) to make us happy? Or is it B) to keep us alive? Yes, it would be nice if you could pick A and B but the right answer is B. The only purpose of food is to keep us alive.

Men only need 2,200 calories a day and women only need 2,000 calories a day to stay alive and healthy. There is not much profit in selling such a small amount of calories a day, so naturally the food industry want us to believe that A is the correct answer. That food makes us happy. Who doesn't want to be happy? If food makes us happy then we have a great reason to eat as much as possible all the time to get as much happiness as possible. More food, more happiness. The food producers want us to overeat. To eat much more than 2,200 or 2,000 calories a day, so they can make more money. But our overeating habits don't bring true happiness but only short bursts of what we call "fake happiness."

Fake happiness is the short sensation of pleasure that we get from the dopamine released in our brain after eating the sugar in Candyfood. We know now that the sugar hijacks our natural hunger cycle and makes us want to eat all the time. The sugar tricks us into feeling fake happiness. The food industry tricks us with marketing to make us believe it's real happiness. Not just real happiness, but the ultimate happiness. They seriously want us to believe the happiness from eating is divine, blissful and heavenly.

The food industry has managed not only to hijack our hunger, but they are also trying to hijacking our happiness by hijacking our definition of happiness. We are being brainwashed by modern food marketing into thinking that food is something "blissful, "divine" and "heavenly." That eating is the new definition of happiness. Think about this. Which other products do you talk about in the way that we talk about food these days? Have you heard people say things like this:

"This pâté is pure bliss."

"Try the cake - it's divine."

"The truffles are to die for."

"I'm in food heaven."

"I live for food!"

"After this dessert I can die happy!"

"I found the meaning of life - it's tiramisu!"

Figure 34

The words we use about food

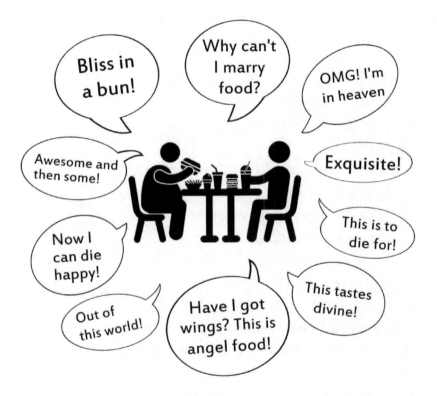

There are so many catchphrases and slogans that we now use almost exclusively use about food experiences. Would you really die for a truffle? Or wish to die after a dessert? Are you really in heaven when you eat? When did we all start talking like this? We used to use those powerful words and phrases about emotions and feelings when we were talking about our family, our children or maybe our faith, but not about a crème friggin' brûlée!

We did a 5-minute online search and it was easy to find many genuine food slogans and taglines from food advertising dating from today and all the way back to the 1950s. Here are a few you might recognize:

I'm Lovin' It
Heavenly crisp Insanely irresistible
Taste the Rainbow
Bounty. The Taste of Paradise
Big. Beefy. Bliss
Baked with love and real ingredients
It'll blow your mind away
Real food for your busy lifestyle
We love to see you smile
What you crave
When you're crazy for chicken
Where the food's the star
A Mars a day helps you work, rest and play
Buy a bucket of chicken and have a barrel of fun
Come hungry. Leave happy
Delicious Food. To fit your lifestyle
Good Mood Food
An oasis of pleasure
We serve passion
Life tastes better with KFC
Making people happy through food
Spur. A Taste For Life
Anything is good if it's made of chocolate
Reward yourself with a Cadbury's Dairy Milk

Comfort in every bar
Don't let hunger happen to you
Get the sensation
Hungry? Why wait?
Makes a Nice Light Snack
Roses grow on you
Sixpence worth of heaven
Do you love anyone enough to give them your last
Rolo?
The sweet you can eat between meals (without ruining
your appetite)

The food advertising people have been trying for years
to turn food into a kind of religion with all their talk of
heaven and angels and floating on clouds of divine bliss
from just a nibble of cake or a spoonful of ice cream.
It's amazing that the great religious prophets didn't
think of this "persuasion" technique. Why all the
sermons and preaching? They could have just handed
out cake! And the Bible could just have been a
cookbook! The 10 commandments could have been 10
Cupcake recipes! New prophets could be called Ben
and Jerry!

Ask yourself these questions: Are the food factories in
heaven? Do angels work in food factories? Can we
really taste heaven? What does bliss taste like? Can you
eat a rainbow? If a bucket of chicken is a barrel of fun
what happens if you buy a barrel of chicken? Do you
get a truck load of fun? And can heaven be sold in
bites? How much is heaven worth in total? A dollar? 10

euro? It's all nonsense! It's marketing gibberish, made up by the "mad men" of the advertising industry.

The food people want us to worship food. They want us to put food up on one of the highest pedestals of our existence - almost at the right hand of God. Move over Jesus; you've been replaced by honey-glazed chicken wings and chocolate-chip ice cream.

The food industry wants to trick us into a lifestyle that has food and eating as its most important part. And it's succeeding. It already succeeded long ago in convincing us that the "kitchen is the most important room in the house." Before food marketing the kitchen was not very important at all. Why is the kitchen now the most important room in the house, when most of us don't even cook anymore? (If you feel like it you can gently slap your hand on your forehead and say Duh!)

Now, you might be thinking to yourself, "No one fooled me - I really enjoy eating! I mean, I'm a foodie! Food is my hobby, it's my life." But ask yourself if perhaps you've been fooled by the food industry into thinking that you love food that much? If you glorify food that much, could it be that you're simply a sugar addict? Could it be that the exposure to a lifetime of marketing and branding has "persuaded" you? What about the hundreds of thousands of ads you've seen of ecstatically happy and slim people smiling and laughing and oohing and aahing when they taste food? Could it be that you have been steered towards a lifestyle of constantly buying and eating more food than you need? Perhaps you were fooled into the Candyfood lifestyle because you've been surrounded with tempting food and now you're constantly responding to the sugar cravings that make you eat when you're not hungry. If you're overweight and love food that much, we think that there's a strong likelihood that you've probably been tricked, and like so many of us, your love of food and your joy of eating gives you mostly "fake happiness" and unwanted extra weight.

We won't go into huge detail about what, in our opinion, the definition of "real happiness" is. (We will have a go at that in a future book, "Stepbac® from Unhappiness.") But we can tell you that, in our opinion, "real happiness" is about living in harmony with nature, other people and yourself. Real happiness comes from loving your family more than food, from being with friends, from living in safety and without fear of illness, and, perhaps most importantly, from good health. And being at a healthy weight is fundamental to good health.

These, in our opinion, are the key elements of "real happiness." We believe that the "fake happiness" that the food advertising is bombarding us with is nothing but sugar-induced sensations of short-term fake happiness, which want to trick you into thinking that you're only happy when you're eating. Fake happiness wears off very suddenly, often to be replaced with unhappy feelings of remorse and regret and, sometimes, physical discomfort when you've overeaten. It's fake happiness, folks.

Look at the next diagram (figure 35).

Figure 35

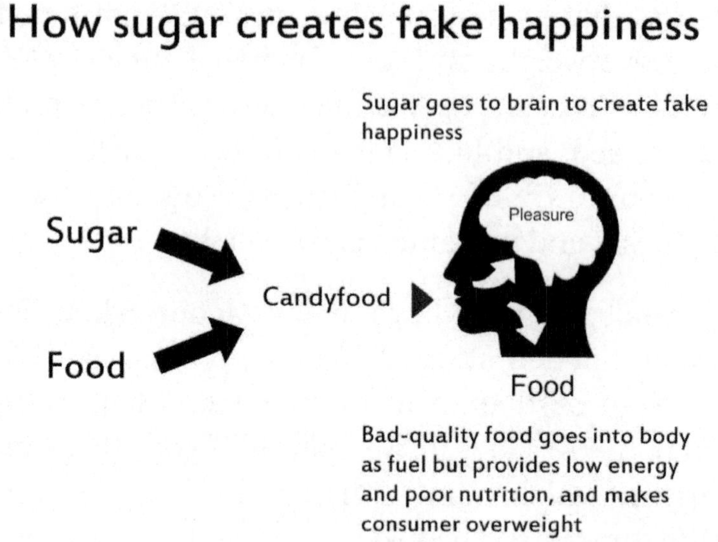

How sugar creates fake happiness

Sugar goes to brain to create fake happiness

Sugar

Food

Candyfood ▶

Pleasure

Food

Bad-quality food goes into body as fuel but provides low energy and poor nutrition, and makes consumer overweight

See how bad-quality food loaded up with sugar works? The sugar goes to the brain. It has no nutritional value but it hijacks your hunger cycle and makes you eat when you aren't hungry. Sugar causes dopamine to be released in your brain which creates short-term "fake happiness" feelings. Sugar creates sugar craving to make you eat again. Fake happiness!

The low-grade food goes to the stomach to be converted into fuel to power your body, but it's low on nutrition so it doesn't give you much energy. Sometimes it even takes more energy to digest bad food than it gives your body back. Oh, and it often makes us overweight. How much bliss is there in that?

Now look at what natural food will do for you (figure 36).

Figure 36

How natural food creates real happiness

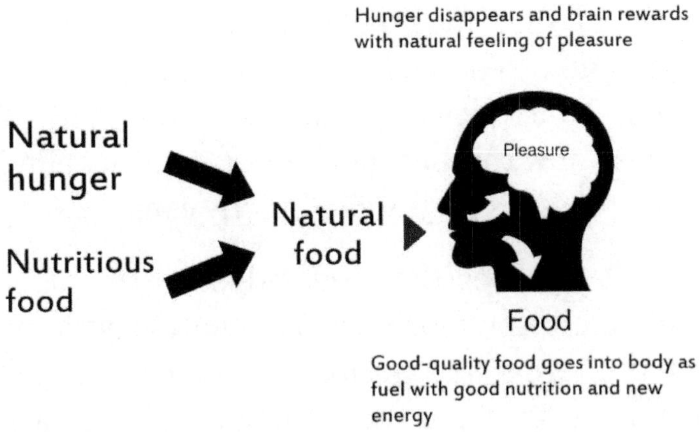

Hunger disappears and brain rewards
with natural feeling of pleasure

Natural
hunger

Nutritious
food

Natural
food

Pleasure

Food

Good-quality food goes into body as
fuel with good nutrition and new
energy

The natural hunger cycle works so that when your body is low on energy it makes you feel hungry. You eat natural food to make the hunger disappear and your brain rewards and thanks you by releasing some dopamine, which makes you feel happy and encourages you to do the same next time you feel hungry. There is no sugar involved in most natural foods. Good-quality food will boost your energy with good nutrition and without causing you to become overweight. That is healthy and good health contributes to real happiness.

Food shopping

When we're at the supermarket, we might assume that we are making our own choices, but is that really the case? The food industry is constantly tricking us in food stores to make us buy more food than we need. Food shopping habits are one of the biggest causes of overeating and being overweight. Simply put, the food industry wants us to "overshop" so it can make more money. When we buy more food we eat more food and the sugar in that food helps keep our fake hunger cravings fully charged. Overshopping leads to overeating which leads to being overweight. Food companies know this but they prefer to turn a blind eye to the health issues they are indirectly causing.

So how exactly does the food industry trick us when we're shopping for food? As we mentioned before, it uses what it terms "persuasion techniques." Many food industry analysts agree that "sneaky tricks" is a more accurate description because the "persuasion techniques" are designed to manipulate us while we're shopping. The food marketing people want to influence our brains into making certain choices while we shop. They want to make us buy something that we did not intend to buy when we entered the supermarket. Is that persuasion - or is it manipulation?

Supermarkets

A little history will help you understand how this started. The food industry began to manufacture processed food on an industrial level in the 1950s and food shopping started to change dramatically. Before then, things like fast food, ready-to-eat meals, TV dinners, frozen food and takeouts did not exist. In those times most people, in many cases housewives (now more appropriately called "homemakers"), did a little food shopping every day.

Most households in Europe did not even have a fridge or a freezer until the 1950s. They might have had an icebox: a small cupboard that looked like a small fridge with a metal box for a big block of ice. Most kitchens had a larder, which was the name for the food cupboard or for a room with food supplies at home. In the larder there was often a marble shelf to keep perishable foods (like milk) a little cooler and keep them fresh for an extra day.

Without a fridge, food could not be stored for long so typically people would visit their local shops on a daily basis. They would take their shopping basket and a shopping list of ingredients to buy the food for the family meals for the next day or two. Shoppers would ask for items at the shop counter and the shopkeeper would measure and weigh food and wrap it for them. Before supermarkets, butcher shops supplied meat, fishmongers sold fish, bakers sold bread and everything else was in a grocer's shop that often also had vegetables.

From the 1960s food shopping started to change dramatically. The Western economies enjoyed an economic boom and with it came modern computer technology, modern marketing methods and supermarkets. Supermarkets offered everything you needed to make meals, but in one big store. The basic idea of a supermarket is to sell everything in one store that previously people bought in many smaller local shops.

Food was cheaper in supermarkets. This was because they bought in bulk and used self-service which meant shoppers would find and collect their own items. This meant lower costs for supermarkets and lower prices for shoppers. That sounds good, but the lower prices meant that shoppers bought more food.

Around the same period, rising standards of living allowed families to move from city apartments into bigger houses in residential suburbs located outside city centers. People in the city moved to the suburbs and people in the country moved there too.

More living space meant bigger kitchens with room for bigger fridges and new inventions like deep freezers. Women entered the workplace more and more, which often meant that in families with children both parents were working. Supermarkets stayed open longer and at weekends so that busy parents could shop outside working hours. All of this meant much less time for daily shopping and for cooking meals with fresh ingredients.

Basically four major changes occurred. One: food shoppers could transport more food in cars; two. shoppers had more food storage space at home in bigger homes with bigger kitchens with fridges and freezers; three: shoppers were making weekly shopping trips by car instead of daily trips on foot or bicycle; four: there was less time to cook meals.

The food companies adapted to these changes; some might say exploited them. They started "helping us" get through modern life by offering us items like "ready-made" food, frozen food and bulk offers.

This all transformed our daily eating and shopping habits completely. "What's wrong with all this," you might ask? "It sounds great. Nobody wants to walk to the shops or cook every day like in the old days." Sure. We agree. It could have been really great! If only supermarkets had "helped us" by just selling us the amount of healthy and natural food that we actually needed to stay at a healthy and natural weight. Now that would have been helpful! Imagine if the food industry had taken a bigger interest in people's health than in its money!

But the food industry is a business. It's not in the business of caring about or helping manage customers' health. It's in the business of making money by selling food. In the early days this new mass food market of supermarkets exploded. It was hugely profitable and billions were earned. This attracted more producers and over time competition grew tough, and so food companies had to use new sneaky marketing methods to make us buy more food so that they could stay ahead of the competition. That is when it started to go wrong. That's when they started tricking us. They didn't mind if the food was healthy. They didn't mind that we were overeating. They didn't care if we were buying more food than we needed, or could even eat. (It is estimated that a third of all food we buy is thrown away!) It's just business. There is not enough profit in selling only the amount of food that healthy people need to eat.

People's health is not what matters, food waste is not what matters - only profits matter.

Even today, when it is safe to assume that all food companies are completely aware of the millions of people who suffer from the misery of being overweight and weight-related illnesses because of unnatural addictions to unhealthy, fake Candyfood, food companies still continue to trick us into buying more food than we need, whenever and wherever they can.

Let's look at some examples of how the food industry tricks us into buying much too much food. In Chapter 6, after we have taught you the Stepbac® from Overeating method, we will give you some tips to avoid being fooled by food marketing tricks.

Bigger shopping baskets and carts

Most people have a shopping list of some kind when they go to the supermarket. What supermarkets want you to do is to wander from your list and buy more things on impulse. One of the ways they help you do this is by making bigger baskets and bigger carts. Scientific studies show that bigger baskets make us buy more. If you have a short shopping list with only a few items on it that you really need, then your items will make a big basket look almost empty, so hey, you feel that you could treat yourself to something more, even though it wasn't on your original shopping list. Some of you might remember the old wire supermarket baskets. You can still find them in small supermarkets or convenience stores. They were tiny and light and without wheels. Shoppers would carry them around the store. In the early days of supermarkets they were in big supermarkets too. We still remember in the 1970s how we carried overflowing wire baskets for our mother with things falling off because the baskets were so small and because we were overshopping.

Before the arrival of hypermarkets, the very big supermarkets, many supermarkets were quite small by modern standards. Many shoppers could walk or cycle to the supermarket and the basket or bag that you used to carry the shopping home in was around the same size as the supermarket wire basket. Today we go by car and supermarket baskets are big and deep and with wheels. Shopping carts are gigantic. Bigger baskets and carts trick us into filling them and buying more (figure 37).

Figure 37

The overshopping evolution

Mr and Mrs Then

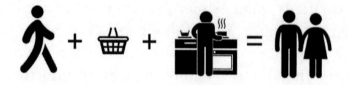

Mr and Mrs Now

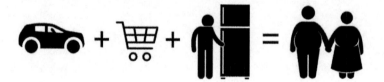

Special offers and impulse buying

Special offers help fill up a big basket or cart. Supermarkets try to manipulate you into buying something on impulse, something that was not on your shopping list, with many special offers. Can you think of anywhere in the world where you get as many great "deals" and "offers" as you do when you're food shopping? These food companies are so generous! So many "gifts"! It's Christmas every day! 20% extra free;

6 packs, 12 packs, 24 packs, 36 packs; 2 for 1, 3 for 2; Limited offer; 50% off second item; Buy one, get one free; Half-price; Family pack, Combo-pack, half-price sale, economy box, best price today. You might have found all the items that were on your original shopping list but there's so much more room in the basket - and so many offers! There's room for a tub of ice cream (it was 2 for 1 and always good to have ice cream, in case someone drops in), a loaf of bread (for a quick snack at home before dinner and anyway it was healthy with full grain and I couldn't resist the fresh smell), a family bag of potato chips with dip for watching a movie after dinner - oh and at the till there was a snack to eat on the way home with the takeaway coffee. Oh Happy Day! Are all these amazing offers really there to help us save money? Are the nice food companies really trying to help us and make our lives easier and better? Are the food companies such lovely and caring people? No. The offers are only there to make us buy more than we need. The offers are there to fool us into buying more.

Many of us don't even check if the price of the offer is actually cheaper. We just assume that it's a good offer but it's not always as cheap as we think. 50% off the second item sounds like you're getting something at half price. But if you buy 2 items then the overall discount is 25% on both. If the offer was "second one free," then it would be 50% percent off. And by the way, as we all know, it is never really "free," if you're buying and paying for it. The limited time offers or the limited number of items are also sneaky tricks. They trick us into thinking that this is such an amazing offer that everyone will want it and that's why there is only a limited number of 3 items per customer. And we buy them thinking, "wow, what a deal!" The truth could be that the store has lots of the "limited time" items on offer in stock. It's more like "unlimited" number of items.

Bulk buying

We are led to believe that bulk buying is cheaper and therefore better. It might be a bit cheaper in the short term and if we buy 24 beers instead of 6 beers or 2 beers then we won't have to buy beer for a month. (Yes it is possible to buy just 2 beers, or even 1 beer!) But what often happens is that when we have more beer in the fridge, then we drink more beer. Then we go back and buy 24 again! It's not really cheaper for you if you consume more beer in a shorter period even if you're paying less per can. Bulk offers like that fool us into buying too much food and drink, and help us to overeat and become or stay overweight.

Free samples or tastings

Free samples. What's not to love about that? Mostly because there's that word "free" again. What other shop gives us so many presents as a food shop? Perhaps supermarkets should be called Santamarkets? But once again a free sample is not really free. Psychological studies have shown that when we are given something, we feel like giving something back. Often when we get a free sample from a nice person, we feel that we should return the gesture and buy one of their products.

Free samples also make shoppers feel excited and a bit special and exclusive because we feel that we got something that not everyone did. That's why the plate of free samples of food is so tiny. To make it exclusive. Free samples are also a cheap way to get shoppers to try something new, which they then might buy - even if it's not on their shopping list.

Supermarket background music

Do you know why supermarkets play slow sleep inducing music? Because slow music makes you walk slowly (like a Food Zombie). Helping you to relax and move slowly means that you have time to notice more things like the special offers - and to buy more. Try wearing headphones playing upbeat fitness music or "Highway to Hell" by AC/DC next time you go shopping and see how it speeds up your shopping and makes you buy less!

Aromas

The big malls and stores often use aromas that are blown from shops or down the aisles to make us feel hungry. Studies show that an aroma of delicious food instantly makes us feel hungry. When we feel hungry, we are more likely to buy more food and we are more inclined to immediately buy some "ready-to-eat" food on impulse to nibble on, rather than only buying the items we went to the mall for. Have you ever eaten or nibbled on the way to the checkout counter? Or on the way to car? Or in the car on the way home?

Some food industry scientists even claim to know which specific smells will make you shop more. Apparently the smell of cinnamon makes shoppers feel a bit weaker and crowded in and this pushes them towards buying more expensive items to compensate for the feeling of weakness. Wow! This is literally "mind blowing" research.

Food placement and supermarket layout

Often the big supermarkets use placement techniques to manipulate us. The expensive high-profit items are at the front of the store, items like fresh food, fruit, fresh bread, etc. The essential items you always need, like milk and water are hidden away somewhere so you have to walk through many aisles and past many items to get to it. The more aisles you walk through looking for something, the more likely you are to be tempted by other products and offers. By the time you find what you're looking for, you might have some impulse items in your basket.

And have you noticed how they move the basics like milk every once in awhile, so you can't ever get too familiar with a big store? And have you wondered why supermarkets don't put up big easy signs, so that you can avoid some aisles and go straight to the section you need? Again it's because they want you to walk through as many aisles as possible. Another sneaky placement trick designed to fool moms into buying candy and snacks for kids is to put some items at kids' eye level so that the kids can grab them and plead for them to go into the basket.

Have you noticed how the fresh and ready-to-go meals - which are usually the most expensive meals - are often just at the entrance of the store? Our local hypermarket here in Barcelona has the fresh sushi just inside. There are several reasons for putting ready meals at the entrance. One is that it makes you hungry immediately. Studies show that if you're hungry, you will buy more food. Another reason is that the profit margin is much higher on ready meals. And it might make you change your mind. Maybe your original shopping list had items for preparing a healthy meal at home but the convenience of a ready meal like rotisserie chicken or pizza is so much easier, that you change your mind and buy a ready meal. That might make you forget the shopping list altogether and you end up coming home without even the one thing on your list that you had actually run out of. Does that sound familiar? So again we are tricked into buying too much and into buying things that we didn't need and into buying overpriced Candyfood. Tricked again.

Price signs

Another food store trick is using misleading price signs and labels. They are everywhere and it's not always easy to understand the offer. Many signs might be also placed so you're not sure which specific product the price or discount refers to. So you take a chance. Haven't we all stood at the checkout and been told that the item we thought was on offer isn't at all, and the offer we saw was for something else? Often we take the item anyway. Tricked again.

Packaging

Ever bought a bigger box of something only to open it at home and find that the box is not full? Tricked again.

Misleading information

Stores might advertise special deals in their promotional material, then when you get to the store the items are already sold out or not there yet because you didn't check the date properly. Tricked again.

Food distribution and availability

Another key part of food marketing is distribution. Nowadays we can get our hands on all kinds of food all day and night. We are surrounded by food. In cities and large towns, it's impossible to go anywhere without being close to food. The food industry surrounds us with food in train stations, gas stations, vending machines, malls, cafés, airports, and on the street. Street food from food trucks is a recent trend in the food industry. Food is everywhere all the time.

Before the 1950s there was simply much less food around. As we told you, people shopped every day and cooked their own meals. They didn't have ready-made snacks. They didn't have fridges. There were no supermarkets, only corner shops. There were no frozen foods. There were no takeouts. In short we were not surrounded by food back then. We didn't walk around eating and drinking on a regular basis. Have a look at how many people walk around with food and drink these days. People in some coastal towns in the United

Kingdom complain of seagulls going "crazy" and attacking humans for their food, which they never used to do. Or perhaps we went crazy. Perhaps we didn't used to eat food outdoors in those towns?

The traditional shopping and eating patterns were based around a natural hunger cycle. There was very little ready-to-eat food and few snacks. Meals had to be prepared. We bought meal ingredients daily in small, local food shops, prepared fresh meals and only ate at mealtimes, when we were hungry (figure 38). All that has changed.

Figure 38

Mr and Mrs Then only ate food at mealtimes

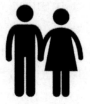

There were very few ready-to-eat meals or snacks. Ingredients for meals were bought on a daily basis from small local food shops

Ingredients were stored at home and only prepared for meals

Most meals were prepared and eaten at home, and there were fewer restaurants

Now we're surrounded by ready-to-eat food all the time - day and night. We buy food much more often. We eat food even when we're not hungry. The sugar makes us hungry all the time and the food industry in developed countries makes sure there is food available to everyone, everywhere and at all times. And if there isn't a physical food outlet near you, you can just order ready-to-eat food via your smartphone. This mass availability of food is also part of the food industry. On top of all its other tricks, the food industry has made sure we are standing knee-deep in food and heading to a future when it is up to our necks and we can never stop eating and never stop feeling hungry (figure 39).

Figure 39

Mr and Mrs Now are surrounded by food all the time

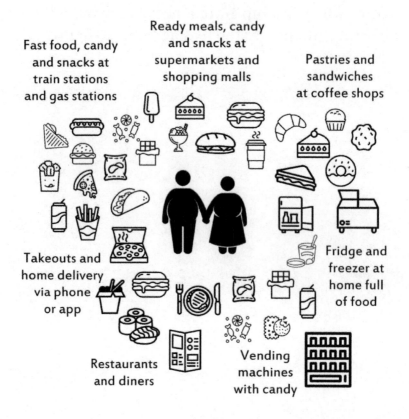

Fast food, candy and snacks at train stations and gas stations

Ready meals, candy and snacks at supermarkets and shopping malls

Pastries and sandwiches at coffee shops

Takeouts and home delivery via phone or app

Fridge and freezer at home full of food

Restaurants and diners

Vending machines with candy

Why is the food industry tricking us? The answer is because they can. The food industry is a business and it does everything it can to make more money. This form of deceptive marketing is not illegal but in our opinion, it should be.

Conclusion: Food marketing chapter

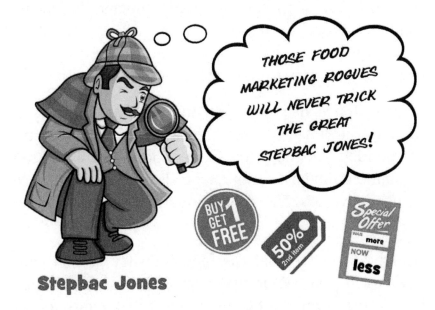

Stepbac Jones

What did Stepbac Jones find out about food marketing? He discovered that the food industry wants to trick us into thinking that eating food is what makes us truly happy. He found out that the short happiness after eating Candyfood is really caused by a sugar rush and that this is fake happiness. Food companies want you to think you're getting a taste of heaven but if you keep tasting their fake heaven it might end up feeling more like hell.

Stepbac Jones found out that the purpose of food advertising is also to constantly remind us that we should keep eating. The added sugar in food is what makes us eat when we're not hungry, but food marketing boosts the sugar addictions by helping to create, reinforce and normalize the many modern habits of overeating that we showed you in the Habits chapter (Chapter 3). Stepbac Jones concluded that the combination of a sugar addiction with many daily unnatural eating habits, is what makes it nearly impossible to stop overeating.

Stepbac Jones also found out that the food industry is tricking us into buying too much food. We are surrounded all day by food. Food is distributed throughout modern society to be always at hand or able to be delivered. The food industry never closes for business.

He found out too that the food industry doesn't care how much you eat or drink or what it does to your health. It is simply a business and it just wants to sell food to make money. The food industry claims that we have a choice about what to buy or eat. No one forces us to buy their products or eat too much. While it is true that they are not forcing us to eat their food by holding a gun to our heads, it is equally true, in our opinion, that they are indirectly forcing us to eat their food by hijacking our natural food habits with sugar. And they are tricking us into overshopping and overeating by influencing us with misleading information. So do we have a real choice if we are being tricked? Or are they indirectly forcing us into eating their fake Candyfood? What do you think?

You now have all the Stepbac® information about the four things that make you want to overeat, which are sugar, habits, cravings and food marketing. As we said at the beginning of this book, the Stepbac® method is the Stepbac® information combined with the Stepbac® action.

So in the next chapter we will teach you what the Stepbac® action is. When you know the Stepbac® action you can use it to Stepbac® from Overeating forever.

Chapter 6

STEPBAC®

ACTION

One thing that will make you stop overeating

AND ABOUT TIME!
I'M READY FOR
SPOT OF ACTION
TO SOLVE THIS
CALORICIOUS CASE!

Stepbac Jones

Chapter 6 – The Stepbac® Action

In the previous chapters you learned about the four things that make you want to overeat, helping you understand why you're constantly overeating. In this chapter we are going to teach you one thing to make you stop overeating. We call this the Stepbac® action.

New non-overeating habit

The Stepbac® action will help you create a new non-overeating habit. In the Habits chapter you learned that you have many different overeating habits with many different triggers to make you automatically feel hungry and want to eat. Among these overeating triggers are sugar cravings, seeing food, smelling food, seeing others eat and having a coffee break, just to name a few of the most common ones.

What we are going to do now is teach you how to change each of your different overeating habits, and how to replace them with one single Stepbac® non-overeating habit. Your new Stepbac® non-overeating habit is simple to learn and easy to remember and use. Look at the next diagram to see how simple it is. The old overeating habit sequence is on the left and the new non-overeating habit is on the right. Notice that in the new non-overeating habit we only change the middle action of the old overeating habit sequence. The trigger and the reward stay the same as in the old overeating habit (figure 40).

Figure 40

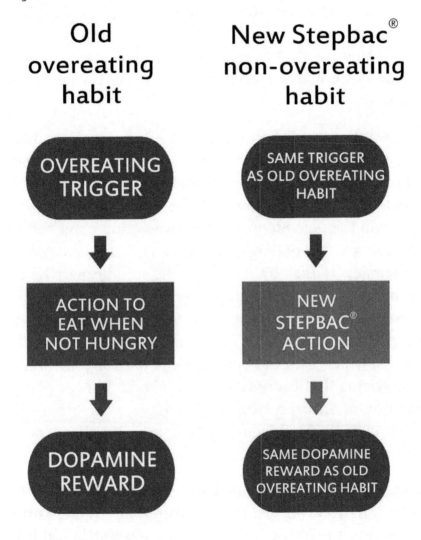

Old overeating habit

OVEREATING TRIGGER

ACTION TO EAT WHEN NOT HUNGRY

DOPAMINE REWARD

New Stepbac® non-overeating habit

SAME TRIGGER AS OLD OVEREATING HABIT

NEW STEPBAC® ACTION

SAME DOPAMINE REWARD AS OLD OVEREATING HABIT

This means that you can change all your current overeating habits by giving them a new middle action. You do not need to learn many new non-overeating habits, only one new action. When you learn the new action you will create one new non-overeating habit that will replace all your old overeating habits. In other words twenty or thirty current overeating habit sequences, that have the middle action of eating when you're not hungry, now become one new Stepbac® non-overeating habit. We will explain what the Stepbac® action is, and how to do it, in a few pages further on in the book.

We want to repeat this concept of creating one new habit to replace all the old ones, because this is very important for you to understand. This is how you will create it. Whenever you feel like having a snack, you must do the new Stepbac® non-overeating habit action instead of the old overeating habit action. What is happening is that by replacing the middle part of all your old overeating habits you're training your brain to learn and store one new non-overeating habit. Your new habit will be stored in the same place as all the old habits, which is in the basal ganglia part of your brain. The goal is that every time you feel fake hunger pangs because of an overeating habit trigger, your brain will automatically load and run the new Stepbac® non-overeating habit sequence.

Here is another diagram that explains again how it works. As you can see, the old overeating trigger is the same. But the old action part of the overeating habit is replaced with a new Stepbac® action. The reward is the same: good old dopamine (figure 41).

Figure 41

New Stepbac®
non-overeating habit

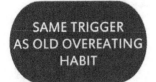

SAME TRIGGER. Could be a typical overeating habit trigger like sugar cravings, smelling food, seeing food, seeing people eat, having a drink, etc.

NEW ACTION. Instead of the old overeating habit action of eating something, you replace that with the new STEPBAC® ACTION

REWARD. The dopamine reward for completing a non-overeating habit sequence stays the same

Look closely at the next diagram to see how you can replace all your overeating habits with one Stepbac® non-overeating habit. Do you see how it works? We modify an old overeating habit to make a new non-overeating habit. An overeating habit with a different middle non-overeating action becomes a new non-overeating habit (figure 42).

Figure 42

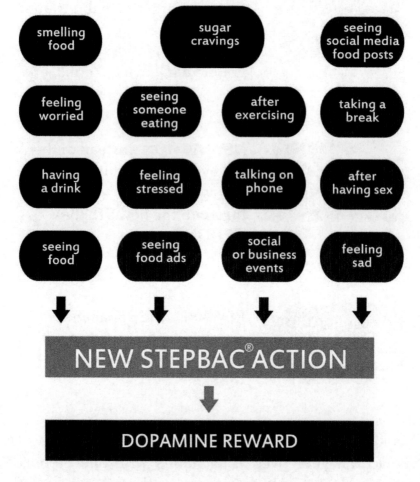

Changing old overeating habits

This is very important. Even though we are sure that you get it by now, let's just repeat it one last time. If we change the middle part of an old habit, then by doing so, we make a new habit (figure 43).

Figure 43

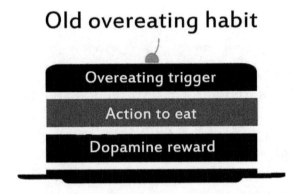

Old overeating habit

Overeating trigger

Action to eat

Dopamine reward

If you put a new middle action in an old overeating habit, it becomes a new non-overeating habit

New non-overeating habit

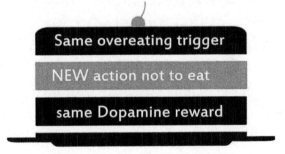

Same overeating trigger

NEW action not to eat

same Dopamine reward

What is the Stepbac® action?

So, finally, it's time. Where is the trumpet fanfare? Now we will tell you what the non-overeating Stepbac® action is and how you must use it to create a new non-overeating habit to replace old overeating habits.

The new Stepbac® action is a physical and mental action, which will make you Stepbac® from overeating and which will help you Stepbac® from buying unhealthy Candyfood when you're food shopping.

You will need a rubber band for the Stepbac® action. Find a rubber band that will fit around your wrist without it feeling too tight. Put the rubber band around your wrist. Left or right wrist is fine. Now we will teach you the Stepbac® action and then, equally important, we will explain in more detail how each part of the Stepbac® action works.

Important! Read this before learning the Stepbac® action

Before we go any further, please understand that the actual Stepbac® action will not work for you unless you have already read Chapters 2-5 with the Stepbac® information about apps, habits and craving. We're going to repeat that to be completely clear: the Stepbac® action only works in combination with the Stepbac® information in Chapters 2-5, it will not work by itself. In other words, you can't skip over the Stepbac® information in this book and only use the Stepbac® action to change your overeating habits. It won't work.

The reason we're telling you this before we teach you the Stepbac® action is because the Stepbac® action is very simple indeed and we don't want you to be disappointed and think, "What? Is that all it is?!" If you were looking forward to reciting a mystical Harry Potteresque formula with closed eyes while clutching your earlobes, well, sorry, but the Stepbac® action is nowhere near as mysterious as that. The Stepbac® action is a simple thing that must be repeated often for a few weeks to create a new habit. It's not something to be done once and then all your habits will be suddenly changed.

The Stepbac® action contains four mental and physical elements, which are neither magic nor unique in themselves but will work because they are very simple. If you have read the previous chapters then you will understand how important it is that the Stepbac® action is not complicated, and that it actually has to be simple. This is because a simple new habit sequence which is repeated many times a day is the key to creating a new habit to replace old smartphone habits. So simplicity is crucial. Simplicity is the "magic." Repeat the simple Stepbac® action many times so your brain will learn and store it as a new habit. It takes a little time and patience, which you must provide. So now let's teach you the Stepbac® action.

The Stepbac® action works like this.

First you take a physical step back, then you snap the rubber band on your wrist, then you say or think to yourself, "Can't Fool Me!" or "CFM." And finally, you smile. While you're doing all these things, which only takes a second or two, you remind yourself of all the ways that you're being tricked into overeating, so that you won't be fooled again into eating when you're not hungry (figure 44).

Figure 44

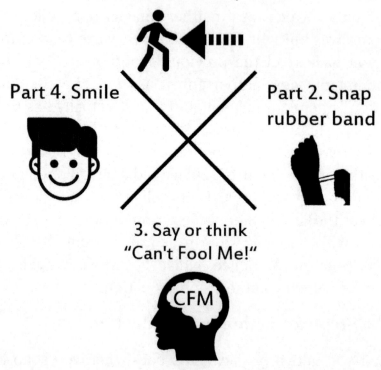

Stepbac® action

Note: You must read Chapters 2-5 first or the Stepbac® action will not work and you will not be able to create a new habit to replace old overeating habits.

Part 1. Take a step back

Part 4. Smile

Part 2. Snap rubber band

3. Say or think "Can't Fool Me!"

CFM

When should you do the Stepbac® action?

You should do it every time you feel fake hunger pangs created by sugar. In Chapter 2 we showed you how sugar hijacks your natural hunger cycle and makes you feel hungry when you are not actually hungry. Those are fake hunger pangs.

How will I know the difference between fake and real hunger pangs?

Good question. The fake and natural hunger pangs feel the same. But it's easy to figure out yourself if you are naturally hungry or "fake-hungry." Basically if you are between meals and have a craving for chocolate, muffins, cake, hotdogs and other sugary Candyfoods, then it's a fake hunger pang created by sugar and you must do the Stepbac® action.

That's it. Are you disappointed that it's so simple? Well, don't be, because simple is good. Simple makes it easy to remember and easy to learn and use. Best of all - it works! We, the writers of this book, have used the Stepbac® action with success to take back control of our eating habits and weight. Remember that you have to repeat this simple Stepbac® action many times to make the habit stick in your brain. Once or twice is not enough. It has to become an automatic reaction to all unnatural feelings of hunger caused by overeating habit triggers.

So let's go into more detail about why we want you to do these specific things in the Stepbac® action. There is a reason for each part of the action and for the

Stepbac® action to work and create the new non-overeating habit, you need to combine the Stepbac® action with the Stepbac® information. Remember this is not a magic formula - you're creating a new habit and need to get it firmly established in your brain, so that it loads and works automatically when you're tempted to overeat. See a muffin - Stepbac® action. Smell a pie - Stepbac® action. See someone eating a donut on TV - Stepbac® action.

Let's look at what actually happens when you do the Stepbac® action. As you can see, the Stepbac® action is a sequence of both physical and mental actions that you do in a fluid sequence that should only take 1-2 seconds. Let's look closer at the Stepbac® action parts one by one.

The Step back

Stepping back is the first part of the Stepbac® action. This is a physical body movement to replace your old physical body movement of eating a snack, overeating at meals and of buying or ordering Candyfood snacks or candy. When an overeating trigger makes you feel "fake hungry" you must physically take a little step backwards - as if to step away from the trigger that is tempting you. This little physical action is enough to replace the old automatic physical action of reaching for food. Think of it as moving away from the food so that you can distance yourself from hunger pangs in the same way that you would step back from something dangerous or unpleasant. Imagine someone holding out a plate of snacks and offering it to you, but instead of taking it you step back so that you physically can't reach it. Imagine yourself in the aisle at the supermarket and seeing a chocolate bar or chips and taking a step back so you just cannot reach them.

The Snap

Snapping your rubber band is the second part of the Stepbac® action. This is also a new physical action to replace your old physical action of overeating. The idea of using a second physical action is to train your brain to make and store this new non-overeating habit. Instead of overeating, the goal is that your brain tells you to automatically step back and then snap your rubber band.

The "Can't Fool Me" (CFM)

Saying or thinking "Can't Fool Me" (CFM) is the third part of the Stepbac® action. This will help to reinforce parts one and two of the Stepbac® action. When you say or visualize the words "Can't Fool Me!" (CFM) you must remind yourself of all the information in this book about the four things that made you want to overeat: Sugar, Habits, Cravings and Food Marketing. You must remind yourself that you do not want to overeat anymore. Remind yourself that your body is no longer a trash can for the food industry. Remind yourself of all the thousands of times that you were fooled into overshopping and overeating by the food industry and all their sneaky "persuasion" tricks and sugared-up fake Candyfood. You must think to yourself that they won't and can't fool you any longer. Ask yourself, am I really hungry - or is this a fake hunger pang? I had a healthy, tasty breakfast and it's not lunchtime yet, so why am I hungry? Ask yourself, do I really need such a big portion? Ask yourself, am I being tricked? Ask yourself, what does my body get from this ice cream? In a few minutes the fake happiness sugar rush will be gone, but I will be carrying 300 calories for a long time. Was I tricked? When you say or think "Can't Fool Me!" (CFM), you will be reminded of the information in this book, and you will be able to break the fake hunger cycle in your brain that was created by sugar. You will be able to Stepbac® and change your old overeating habits. If you prefer, you can also just choose to say or think the initials of "Can't Fool Me!", which are CFM.

The Smile

A smile is the fourth part of the Stepbac® action. After stepping back, snapping your wrist band and saying "Can't Fool Me" or "CFM," remember always to smile. Force a smile if it does not come by itself. The smile is another physical action and an important one. Smile because you're happy that you didn't eat that snack or didn't buy a snack or eat too much at a mealtime. Smile because you now know they won't be able trick you ever again. Smile because you have taken back control of your own brain and body. You are in control again, not the food companies. Smile because you feel great about being a natural eater again. Smiling will reinforce your achievement of not giving in to a fake hunger feeling. It will strengthen your new non-overeating habit of stepping back physically and mentally from the action of overeating in all its forms. Smiling will make you feel good and happy, and is your reward for learning and using your new Stepbac® non-overeating habit. Did you know that when you smile even a forced smile your brain will naturally release a little bit of dopamine that will make you feel a bit happy, helping reduce the need for a dopamine hit from sugar. Smiling means you get the same dopamine reward as you would have got from the sugar. But now you're getting it without overeating and without opening your body to unwanted weight. You're breaking the fake hunger survival cycle in your brain.

So the physical and mental Stepbac® action with its four parts is designed to remind you of everything you have learned in this book about sugar, habits, cravings and marketing. Your new Stepbac® action will quickly start to create a new non-overeating habit sequence. By doing it you will train your brain to store your new Stepbac® non-overeating habit sequence and to load it whenever you experience an overeating trigger. Take a Stepbac® from overeating and you will be taking back control of what goes in your body. You will have stepped back to your life as it was before you were "taken" by the food industry.

What if you can't take a physical step back? Well, depending on where you are, it's no problem to vary the Stepbac® action a little bit. If you're sitting down, then you can't very well take a step back, but you could try sitting back in your chair or sitting more upright in your chair. If you're standing then, instead of stepping back, you could clasp your hands behind your back and put one hand over your rubber band. You can't eat very well with your hands behind your back.

But please remember, you must always do something Stepbac® related when you encounter overeating triggers or cravings to help train your brain into accepting that you don't want to eat now. Keep doing it. Repetition is key to forming a new habit. It's especially important in the first hours and days after deciding to stop overeating that you always use all four parts of the Stepbac® action sequence: take a Stepbac®, snap your rubber band, say or think "Can't Fool Me!" (or "CFM") and smile!

Don't feel embarrassed about doing this. Don't think it's childish or silly. The Stepbac® method works and there is nothing embarrassing about using a method to change overeating habits. The Stepbac® doesn't have to be very obvious. A little step back is fine; you don't have to strain a muscle or set a record. No one will notice that you snap your rubber band or quietly say to yourself "Can't Fool Me!" And anyway, who cares what people think? It's a free world. You want to stop overeating and take back control of your eating, and this is how to do it. So this is about you and no one else. Do the Stepbac® action every time you feel an overeating habit trigger, or a fake hunger pang or craving and you will be able to stop overeating for good and get back to natural eating habits.

What will happen after you stop overeating?

Any sugar withdrawal symptoms and cravings are strongest during the first days after you decide to stop overeating. That is because your brain is all fired up by sugar. You're riding the sugar bus at full speed on the sugar highway. The fake hunger survival cycle and the many overeating habits are driving the bus. You are just a passenger.

After you stop overeating, then your power over sugar addiction and Candyfood marketing will quickly grow stronger. Not as quickly as the Incredible Hulk, but your power will grow stronger while the power of sugar will quickly grow weaker. (If you turn green like the Incredible Hulk, see a doctor.)

After you start to use the Stepbac® method, your sugar cravings will weaken as you Stepbac® from them. Visualize that you're stepping back further and further from sugar and Candyfood. The sugar cravings will become weaker and smaller and soon they will wither and die. They will be a speck on the horizon and finally a distant memory.

After a week it will start to feel like the sugar addiction gave up the fight and disappeared to find another body to trash. You will probably be surprised at how quickly your new Stepbac® non-overeating habit will start to give you the upper hand. With every Stepbac® you take, you grow stronger and the fake hunger pangs grow weaker. The distance will seem to become longer and longer between you and all the Candyfood that you used to crave. It will almost feel like you moved back in time and are once again becoming the non-overeating person that you once were in childhood before you started to overeat and snack all the time. When you start to feel sugar has lost its power over you and you are using your new Stepbac® action to defuse the old overeating habits, you will really know that you're back in control of your eating habits. Look at the next diagram, the Stepbac® action pyramid. This is what will happen (figure 45).

Figure 45

Stepbac® action pyramid

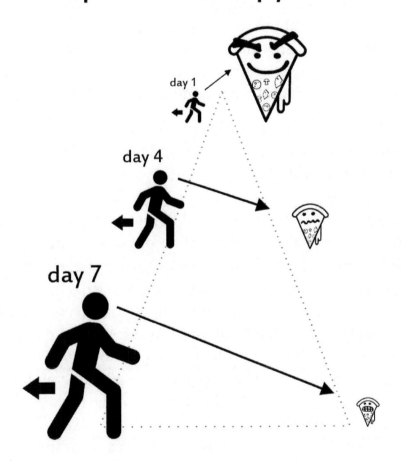

Try the Stepbac® action now

Practice the Stepbac® action right now. Stand up, take a little step backwards, snap your rubber band, then think or say "Can't Fool Me!" or "CFM!" And smile. Every time you do this you're actively creating, practicing and strengthening your new non-overeating habit. This new single Stepbac® non-overeating habit is what you will use to replace all your old overeating habits. The physical and mental action sequence will remind you of everything you have read in this book about sugar, about overeating habits and cravings, about triggers and about food marketing. Practice the Stepbac® action again. Keep doing it until it's an automatic habit and you can do it without thinking.

Let's talk a little more about the hours and days after you decide to stop overeating. There will be physical effects like withdrawal symptoms and fake hunger pangs. You will feel them for a few days because the sugar levels in your body will be dropping. First of all you should know that the physical withdrawal symptoms are small and weak and nowhere near as bad as you think. Fake hunger pangs are like a feeling of emptiness in your chest or stomach. You really think you feel hungry. You think you want to eat. But don't be fooled. Stepbac® from them. You are not hungry. You don't need to eat. These sugar withdrawal symptoms will come and go a bit for the first few days as you adjust to your new life of not overeating. There is no real pain from hunger pangs or sugar withdrawal symptoms, only brief annoyance and discomfort, but this will quickly get smaller and smaller and you will be able to suppress and conquer this annoyance and discomfort. Later when you have stepped back from fake hunger, you will know when you really are hungry. Actually you might be surprised at how seldom you feel hungry. We humans only need 2,000-2,200 calories daily in a balanced food plan to be healthy, and to be honest it's not hard to reach that number so you probably won't feel hungry very often. When you reach that point you will fully understand how it was fake hunger prompting you to eat.

It is unavoidable that you will experience some sugar withdrawal symptoms when you start to take a Stepbac® from Candyfood. You might also find that your sleep patterns are a bit different and you might feel a little more tired than usual. Any changes that you feel are completely normal and are just signals that your body is adapting to this big interior spring clean. The sugar cravings will be worst during the first days after deciding to stop overeating because there is still sugar in your system and all your overeating habits are active. Already by the fourth day both will be weaker. After one week you will probably be very surprised at how little they affect you and you will start to feel that you have taken back control. This moment is when it's most important to keep doing the Stepbac® action. Don't celebrate victory too early, even if you hardly feel any fake hunger pangs. Don't think that you can just turn a sugar addiction on and off like a tap. That will not work. You can't eat many sugary snacks one day and then just Stepbac® on the next day. That will mean that you're constantly fighting strong cravings and bad eating habits. It is better to aim to remove unnatural sugar from your food intake and keep it that way. The reason for this is that sugar is addictive and it will pull you back into the Candyfood lifestyle if you don't keep stepping further and further back. Just a snack or two a day and you risk your natural hunger survival cycle being hijacked again by sugar. So don't let the sugar terrorist back into the cockpit of your brain.

The most critical time to use the Stepbac® action is the first week, but make sure you keep taking a Stepbac® many times a day for the first three weeks and even longer. We the authors still Stepbac® from snacks many times a day because it has become a habit. We live in Barcelona, Spain so, for example, we see many tourists eating ice creams and gelatos, but we automatically Stepbac® and very rarely order them ourselves. We are in control and we choose energy, health and real happiness over a 3-minute sugar rush of fake happiness with 300 useless calories that we would have to carry around in the hot sun! Believe in the Stepbac® method. When you feel sugar cravings or fake hunger pangs or when you feel the pull of familiar overeating habit triggers trying to make you cave in and have a gelato, use the Stepbac® action to step back from them. It will work!

You might be surprised at how many times you find yourself taking a Stepbac® in the days after you decide to stop overeating. With your new-found knowledge of sugar habits, cravings and food marketing you will now see clearly how your "old" life was a minefield of overeating triggers: colleagues overeating, people outside cafés overeating, coffee breaks with unnecessary snacks, cravings to overeat candy after dinner, seeing people overeat on TV and in movies, and so on. All these overeating habit triggers try to make you overeat. You need to fight them by using your new Stepbac® action.

Practice your new Stepbac® action again a few times, so you're ready to use it. Think of an overeating trigger such as being in a coffee shop, and practice your new Stepbac® action so that you don't order or eat your "favorite" snack. Remember that you need to keep doing this for the coming weeks until it becomes an automatic habit in your brain. Your old overeating habits are dying, but they are not dead. So keep using the Stepbac® action to create your new non-overeating habit, which will take over more and more from all the old overeating habits. The more time passes, the more motivated you will be, as you start to enjoy your new overeating-free life without having to think or worry about food or eating all day long.

Over a period of just a few weeks, your brain will have created and stored the new Stepbac® non-overeating habit. By then, when you see overeating triggers you will stop thinking about them, because you will have created the new Stepbac® non-overeating habit that will automatically reject the overeating trigger by reminding your subconscious that you won't be fooled into eating when you're not hungry or into overeating. As soon as your new non-overeating habit is stored in your brain permanently then you won't miss overeating at all, because the new non-overeating habit will kill the cravings too. After months and years you will actually probably wonder how you could so easily have been fooled into eating all the time. You will feel like you have control of your food and not that your food controls you. You will visit supermarkets and walk through the candy section and ice cream section and not even think about reaching for any of it. You will know that at least 75% of the food in modern supermarkets is Candyfood and full of sugar, and you just won't want it in your body. You will be back in control of your body.

Conclusion: Stepbac® action chapter

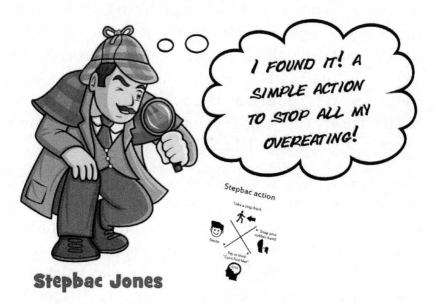

Stepbac Jones

What did Stepbac Jones learn in the Stepbac® action chapter? He discovered that you can change all your former overeating habit sequences into one single new non-overeating habit sequence. To do this, every time you feel an overeating trigger you must use the Stepbac® action of taking a step back from Candyfood, then snapping a rubber band on your wrist to remind you of the Stepbac® information, then saying or thinking "Can't Fool Me!" or "CFM," and smiling. Doing this action will defuse each old overeating habit and make it into a nice new non-overeating habit.

He found out that the fake hunger pangs will disappear as the sugar loses its grip on your natural hunger cycle and you won't want to eat when you're not hungry. Now you will only want to eat when you really are naturally hungry, which is usually at mealtimes because we only need 2,000-2,200 calories a day to power our bodies. If we get these calories we don't feel hungry very often.

Well done for finishing this chapter and practicing the Stepbac® action. In the next chapter we will give you some tips to help you prepare for your new life as a Stepbaccer.

Chapter 7

STEPBACCER TIPS!

Some inspiration and support for your new life as a Stepbaccer!

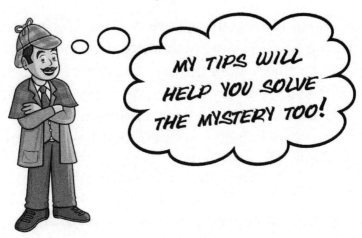

Stepbac Jones

Chapter 7 - Tips for being a Stepbaccer

When you start using the Stepbac® action and the Stepbac® method, you will start to change your overeating habits to natural eating habits. As you now know the goal is to replace all your bad food shopping habits and overeating habits with one new good habit of taking a Stepbac® from buying and overeating food that your body doesn't need. This could be a major change in your daily life and lifestyle, so here are some tips from the authors to help you make your new Stepbac® lifestyle a success.

Count calories

It's essential to count calories. Most food items these days have a food label with nutrition content where you can see calorie amounts, so it's easy to keep count of the calories you eat during the day. Start thinking about how to eat smaller portions of healthier food. Make a simple daily meal plan that has the same basic types of meals every day.

Think of it like this: a healthy pet normally eats the same food in the same amounts every day, and even from the same bowl. Occasionally a pet gets a treat but most pet owners know that the best way to keep a pet healthy is to feed it the right amount of nutritious pet food every day. Keep that in mind. We humans are animals too. We should adopt the same approach to our daily meals if we want to be healthy.

Obviously we are not suggesting that we start eating pet food, but we should aim to follow a similar meal plan. We should eat basic, healthy meals in a healthy amount every day. Of course for a special occasion we could enjoy a slightly bigger meal or a treat but our day-to-day food should always be a simple, balanced mix of food in the right amounts. You could make your own collection of meal recipes which you can rotate so it does not get as repetitive as pet food, but it is important that you eat the same basic meals every day in the right amounts. That way you know you're getting the right amount of calories and a healthy mix of nutrients. Remember always that the reason we eat is to power our body, not to make us happy. Eat for fuel, not for fun!

As we have said several times, Stepbac® is not a weight-loss diet, but Stepbac® can be a very important tool in your life to help you take back control of what you put in your body. Using the Stepbac® method you will find it easier to eat less and to stop overeating unhealthy food. Stepbac® can be used to stop gaining weight - or to lose weight.

Here's how using Stepbac® can help you stop weight gain or for weight loss. As we have mentioned, the average amount of energy from food that we need to fuel our body is 2,200 calories for men and 2,000 calories for women. This is an average, so check your own daily calorie need online by searching for a Calorie Calculator.

To stay at the same weight

To stop weight gain and to stay at the same weight that you are now, then you should only eat the number of calories that your body needs per day to power your body. If you eat the right amount then you will not gain weight - or lose weight. For example, if you're an average male and you weigh say 90 kg/200 lbs then you need to eat around 2,200 calories each day. If you do this, then your body weight will stay at 90 kg/200 lbs. If you eat more calories in one day than the 2,200 calories than your body needs for the day, then you will gain weight on that day.

To lose weight

To lose weight you have to eat fewer calories than your body needs per day. So if you're an average male who needs 2,200 calories per day, then you must eat fewer than the 2,200 calories a day that your body needs if you want to lose weight. Generally it is considered that you could safely eat 500 calories less per day than your recommended average to achieve weight loss. Very low-calorie food plans should be avoided in our opinion and should always be monitored by a medical professional. Remember when you're trying to lose weight that it's very important that you understand it is not healthy or safe to starve yourself or stop eating entirely even for a short period to lose weight. Your body must have energy from food to function and it cannot function without food. And there is a limit to how few calories you can consume a day, which means that weight loss is always a gradual process. The most weight one can safely lose is estimated by experts to be around 1 to 2 lbs per week (450 to 900 grams) which is ¼ to ⅓ lb (113.5 to 150 grams) per day. Safe, healthy weight loss can only be gradual so be patient. Get into the Stepbac® lifestyle and you will be in control of your eating and can plan your weight loss or stay at your current weight.

When considering a daily food plan also remember that your daily calories must come from varied sources and you must always eat a balanced mix of healthy foods with the necessary nutrients of carbohydrates, proteins, fats, vitamins and minerals. Search online and you will find plenty of webpages with suggestions for making food plans and which healthy foods to include - or, even better, consult a dietician and ask them to make a food plan for you.

Daily physical activity

When you use Stepbac® to stop overeating, then for those people who are only a few pounds overweight, just half-an-hour of moderate physical activity a day is enough to either maintain your weight or help you lose weight. Many people think getting exercise means joining a gym or jogging. That's wrong. All movement and activity burns calories and even small movements will help your body function much more efficiently and improve both physical and mental health. If your goal is to lose as much weight as is safely possible per day, then of course a little more daily physical activity in a gym or doing sports will speed up your weight loss. But it's important to understand that you can easily get a daily half hour of physical activity without being a triathlete or half-marathon runner.

There is plenty of movement in changing small daily habits. For example, you could park your car a little further from the supermarket entrance and walk the last bit. Or park it on the lowest level of an underground car park and walk up the steps. You could buy less and carry it to the car instead of in a trolley. Why not get off the bus at an earlier stop and walk the rest of the way home? Or cycle the first part of the commute to work and then catch the train or bus the rest of the way. Stop using the bus stop nearest to your home but instead walk to the second nearest stop and catch the bus there. Get off the elevator one or two floors early at the office and walk up the last floors. Take the steps instead of escalators. Play with your children outside or go for a walk with them instead of playing computer games. Go for a fifteen-minute walk after lunch and dinner. Tidy the house or polish the car windows. There are many small ways to move your body which all burn calories. Where will I get the energy from for all that you might think? When you Stepbac® from Overeating you will soon feel the energy of your youth flowing back to your body, so use it to get your body moving more and more every day.

Reevaluate your "favorite" food

Most of us have favorite foods. Something we "can't live without!" or "would kill for" or "die for!" It's all very dramatic (thanks food marketing people for turning food into Shakespearean dramas!). If you're going to change your overeating habits then you might have to say goodbye to some of your favorite things. Your favorite dishes or brands could be sugar bombs that will keep sabotaging your Stepbac® lifestyle. We recommend that you check out how much sugar and how many calories you're dumping in your body when you eat your favorite food or snacks. Then decide how to limit eating them or just take a big Stepbac® and ditch them altogether. We, the authors of "Stepbac® from Overeating," used to "love" barbeque spare ribs and we had a favorite ribs restaurant in Barcelona. We used to have ribs at least once a month, but after using the Stepbac® method we only have ribs once a year. At the time of writing it's been at least 8 months. It's just too big a meal, too big a portion, and after becoming used to the Stepbac® lifestyle, a big rack of ribs with a side order of fries and coleslaw just makes us both feel much too full and takes too long to digest. Stepbac® made us change our attitude to our favorite food and now we don't crave ribs anymore or miss them. Maybe Stepbac® will do the same for you and your favorite comfort food.

Only eat at regular mealtimes

When you start to Stepbac® you will be buying less food and be eating fewer snacks. You often hear people suggest that one should replace unhealthy snacks with healthy ones. But when you use Stepbac® you will probably not feel the need to eat snacks; using Stepbac® stops you from feeling hungry all the time which means that you don't really feel the need to snack between meals. What will happen is that you will think less about eating in general and you will simply look forward to your regular meals like breakfast, lunch and dinner. If you eat balanced regular meals then you should not feel real hunger very often, but if you do, then it is a healthy sign that your natural hunger process is back to normal and your body is giving you a hint that you need to top up your energy in the form of healthy calories. So focus on eating only at your regular mealtimes and don't mess up your natural hunger cycle with many between-meal snacks. Try not to have snacks on your desk or in your fridge. And consider drinking more water between meals.

Demote your kitchen

Remember how the food industry wants your kitchen to be the "most important room in the house"? Well, it also wants your fridge to be a brightly lit "home-supermarket" display so that you can see an alluring display of colors, packaging and choices to tempt you into overeating when you open your fridge. It wants your freezer to be a "home-supermarket" storage unit always stocked up with ready- to-heat/eat food. Maybe it's time to take a Stepbac® from spending too much time in your kitchen. Maybe it's time to demote your kitchen to the "least important room in the house." Turn it back into the room that it was at the start of the last century: a place where meals are prepared and only fresh food is stored instead of it being the kind of "Food Adventure" theme park that modern kitchens have become. Consider getting a smaller fridge and freezer.

Or block off some shelves in the fridge so you can't fill it up with as much food. Limit your choices. Just buy and store what you need for a day or two of healthy eating. Consider also cutting down on cooking appliances so your kitchen is not an in-house fast food outlet, where you can make all kinds of "calorific" fast food yourself. Don't be fooled by the food marketing that "food is fun." Food is fuel. Good health is fun!

Food shopping

If possible go shopping more often but only buy the items on your shopping list. Get what you need for a day or two, so that you don't fill your fridge and freezer. No food at home means less snacking and overeating. You won't overeat if there's no food. Use Stepbac® and you won't buy all the fake Candyfood that you used to buy at the supermarket, plus you won't be distracted and fooled by offers and tricks when you shop for food. When you're at the till, check the items in your basket or trolley and if you spot something that ended up in the basket in a weak moment (it can easily happen in the early days of starting to use Stepbac®), then you can always take a Stepbac® at the till and take it out of the basket or trolley again.

Avoid supermarket deals

Avoid supermarket deals and "gifts" in general, unless perhaps it is something that was on your shopping list and that you need. But be careful of being fooled into stocking up on a food item that will then sit in your fridge and make you overeat. Most bulk special offers want you to buy more so that you eat more. Avoid the free samples completely. They will just make you hungry between meals.

Speed shop

Speed up your food shopping. Check what time you go in to the supermarket and try to be out again as quickly as possible - without knocking over any shoppers or displays, of course! Speed shopping habits will help reduce temptation as you start using Stepbac®. When you have established your daily food plan and the Stepbac® habit is automatic, then you will be able to quickly walk through a supermarket and only choose the food you need. You might be surprised at how little you want to buy in big supermarkets. 90% percent of modern-day food is Candyfood and you will no longer want to buy or eat it. You will be a Stepbaccer.

Consider using a dietician

You don't have to consult a dietician. We, the authors, have never talked to a dietician. There are many websites with free advice about making food plans, recipes for healthy meals, and portion sizes written by excellent dieticians and medical experts, but if you feel you have no idea about how to prepare or eat natural and healthy food and you don't have time to check out many blogs and websites, then by all means find a local dietician and ask him/her to help prepare a personal food plan with natural eating habits and regular meals. Remember Stepbac® is not a diet in itself. It's a tool to help you change your overeating and overshopping habits.

Social functions

What if most of your family is a bit overweight and not really into a healthy lifestyle? How do you Stepbac® from overeating when everyone around you is eating all day and trying to tempt you back into their lifestyle? Here's how. Tell your friends and family that you have decided to improve your health and take a Stepbac® from unhealthy food and snacks. No one will blame you for being a Stepbaccer. Tell them about the book. Tell them how much better you feel now that you control what goes into your own body. Become a Stepbaccer and spread the word, but don't bully anyone or pity them or shame them. People should be allowed to live their own lives and make their own choices. If they ask you for advice, then by all means, explain how Stepbac® works but it's very difficult to explain the method in just a few words so it's better to suggest they read the "Stepbac® from Overeating" book themselves.

Be patient

Remember Stepbac® is not a diet but a tool to help you change your overeating habits and lifestyle. When you have learned to Stepbac® it can help you on a journey back to your natural weight, but this could well take months or even years depending on how much you weigh and how fast you want to lose weight. You can decide the pace but if you use Stepbac® you will find it easier to achieve your weight goal, which is to reach and stay at your natural weight. Along the journey, by using the Stepbac® method you will quickly start to feel healthier, happier and more energized, and you will know that you will be able to reach your natural weight. Remember to always avoid extreme low-calorie food plans and consult a medical professional if you're very overweight.

Re-read the book

Re-read "Stepbac® from Overeating." Keep it handy and check chapters to refresh your memory about how sugar tricks people into overeating. Use the Stepbac® action you have learned and you will soon enjoy your new healthier lifestyle; you will slowly but surely start to see the results of your Stepbac® from overeating. We welcome you to visit us at www.stepbac.com to find tips and inspiration and to help inspire others.

What not to do

DON'T use Stepbac® as a short-term diet

The Stepbac® method is not a short-term weight-loss diet. Short-term diets have been around since the 1970s and they don't work for most people in the long term. Think about why they don't work. If you're overweight because of unhealthy eating habits, and then you diet for a short period of time and lose weight, then the diet would work if you changed your lifestyle. But if you go back to the same unhealthy lifestyle after the diet, which most people do, then of course the diet will not work in the long term.

Do not try to use Stepbac® as a weight-loss diet or as a way to stop eating for a short period. Stepbac® is not a short- or a long-term diet plan. The Stepbac® method is a way to change your overeating habits into natural eating habits. Stepbac® is a tool that you can use to defend yourself against the many sneaky food tricks that the food industry uses to fool you into overeating when you're not hungry. If you use Stepbac® then you can control what you eat. This means that you can use Stepbac® to either stop weight gain or to lose weight and get back to a healthy weight.

DON'T set a date for a weight

Don't set a date to reach a certain weight. Many people set themselves a challenge to slim down to a specific weight to look their best for a wedding or a bikini vacation. We don't think that's a good idea. Why mess with your weight just for the sake of a wedding photo or a bikini size? Go to your weddings and parties at the weight you are on the day. The same applies to vacations. Dates are not important. Your family and friends will not care if you're a bit overweight on a certain date. What they care about is having you in their lives for a long time as a happy and healthy person! So don't ever feel pressured to set a date for a weight. Learn the Stepbac® from Overeating method and have patience. You will take back control of your weight - one Stepbac® at a time!

DON'T aim for "six-pack" abs or a "bikini-ready" body

Don't be fooled by fitness magazines and photoshopped bikini models. Having a six-pack or a bikini model figure is an over-hyped illusion of fake happiness. Of course, if you want to participate in Mr Universe competitions then by all means go get a six-pack from daily workouts and strict diets. But remember that most people never had a six-pack, don't need a six-pack and will never work as models. Don't be fooled by glossy magazines and gossip websites. We regular types can look healthy, slim and fabulous without killing ourselves in the gym and without hyped-up celebrity diet fads. Use Stepbac® to gradually reach your natural weight by not overeating and then get a sensible amount of daily exercise.

DON'T feel deprived

Don't feel miserable. Don't feel you're being deprived of something magical when you stop overeating. Don't be fooled into thinking food makes you happy! Don't feel that you have been locked alone outside the Food Adventure theme park while everyone else is inside enjoying life and feeling happy! It's the other way round - never forget that! As we've shown you, food is not the meaning of life. Food is not the foundation of happiness. Health is the foundation of happiness. Food is only fuel for your body to stay healthy so that you can enjoy every day of a long and healthy life. You will still enjoy delicious food, but just not all the time or in unnatural amounts. When you take the first Stepbac®

to control what you eat, you will still be surrounded by food marketing tricks every day. You will still notice how people around you are overeating. They are snacking, having seconds, piling food on their plates. They might be tempting you with it. "Come on... one little bite. Join us. Be like us." All that pressure will not disappear from your life. But you can make it disappear from your mind. Use the Stepbac® action that you have learned to remind yourself that many people have been "taken" by the food industry. They are "slaves" to food. They are trapped in overeating habits that seduce them and trick them with fake happiness. Many people might spend most of their lives either miserably dieting or miserably wishing they could lose weight. When you're able to take back control of what you eat and control your weight then you will not feel miserable. You will feel happy. You will not have found the "meaning of life." You will still have ups and downs, and daily problems. Of course you will. We, the authors, have plenty of daily problems and we don't know what the "meaning of life" is either, but at least by using Stepbac® you will know fake Candyfood from real food and fake happiness from real happiness, and one thing's for sure: overeating will no longer be the fake meaning of your life.

DON'T become a bore, bully or fanatic

Be a Stepbaccer but don't turn into a bore, bully or fanatic. By this we mean that just because you have read this book and have started to change your overeating habits, that doesn't give you the right to start preaching to friends and family and criticizing their overeating habits or bullying them into eating what you think they should eat. Believe us, nobody likes unwanted advice and it will probably lead to tension in your social relationships. Just focus on your own life and mind your own Stepbac® business. When you're able to control your weight and your energy starts rising, then friends and family will probably ask how you're doing it and then you can share your new knowledge by recommending that they read this book. But don't preach, teach, bully or lecture everyone around you about how they are being tricked by the food industry, that they don't get real happiness from eating a cake, or that they have lost control of their lives, blah blah blah. People need to be allowed to live their own lives and to make their own choices. You made a personal choice to read this book to help you make changes in your own life because you felt unhappy with your weight. Let others make a similar choice themselves when they feel that the time is right for them.

DON'T be bullied into overeating

Don't let yourself be bullied. When you choose to exchange your old overeating habits with a new Stepbac® eating habit, then you might be the first in your community or family to make such a change of lifestyle and this could bring many challenges in your social circles. A lot of social contact these days seems to involve cooking, eating or drinking. Some people might feel bad about themselves when you seem to be able to

Stepbac® from Overeating with such little effort. Some people might want to have a snack but if you say "no thanks" to joining them, they might be resentful of your Stepbac® "superpower" and chastise or bully you. We, the authors, have been told by family members we were "antisocial" and "undernourished fanatics" after we started eating less. We still get comments like "oh yeah, I forgot you only eat air" and it's "not normal to eat that little." If you experience this then tell them gently that they are welcome to eat whatever and whenever they want and in return could they kindly respect your choice to not overeat.

DON'T change your life to avoid food

Don't try to avoid food, or avoid meeting certain people or being in certain situations. There is no need to avoid a party or celebration where you know there will be a free buffet or free drinks. Don't try to avoid certain people because you think they will have a bad influence on your new Stepbac® eating habits. On the contrary, enjoy your new life and enjoy the great social events that life pushes your way. Simply use your new Stepbac® action to take control of these situations, so that you decide and control what you eat and drink. You can still treat yourself to a piece of cake on special occasions if you want to, of course you can. But as you're now in control of your eating habits you can choose to take one piece of cake - rather than taking two pieces as you might have done in the pre-Stepbac® days. Once you have understood and learnt the Stepbac® method, then you will feel confident that you really can enjoy yourself on your own terms and regulate your eating habits.

Chapter 8

YOU CAN DO IT!

A pep talk from the authors

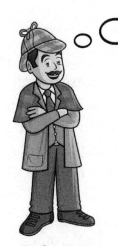

MMM..
I WONDER WHY
IT'S CALLED
A PEP TALK?

Stepbac Jones

Chapter 8 - You can do it!

Well done! Just a few more pages and you will have finished this book. This last chapter is a "pep talk" from the authors, Carl and Peter.

You probably know that a "pep talk" is a talk that someone gives to encourage another person/or themselves. For example, a coach gives his team a pep talk before a game. To give a pep talk means to give a short speech to give encouragement, confidence, enthusiasm and to energize the listener(s) to make them believe in their heart and soul that they can truly achieve something great. The basic message of a pep-talk message is: "You can do it!"

But did you know that the origin of the word "pep" is from the spice pepper? This is because pepper adds energy and spice to food. To "pep up" means to boost something or someone with energy and spice. Over time, people started using the word in the expression "a pep talk." For us that's just the perfect way to end this book. What better way to give you the courage, confidence and energy to get sugar out of your life than with a pep talk to help convince you that you can do it!

The reason we want to give you our pep talk is because we think you might feel a little nervous or worried that you might not be able to do this. That Stepbac® might not work for you or you won't learn it. Don't worry! It will work. It's easy to learn and use. Don't feel scared. We know you can do it!

Sometimes a pep talk has a little bit of something to make you feel just a little indignant or, even a little bit mad. Like... hey... they fooled me a lot in the past but they cannot fool me again! Here's an interesting thing about the food industry and its sugar scam that most people don't really notice and which might make you feel indignant. Not only does the food industry try to fool you all the time. But who takes the blame and who feels guilty about weight gain? You do! It's almost the "perfect crime!" They trick you and make you overweight, but you blame yourself and your lack of willpower. You blame yourself, not the food industry. What a perfect scam!

Imagine if someone robbed a bank and the bank blamed itself instead of the crooks. That's what's happening here. They trick you so you put on weight, then you take the blame and feel bad! Well, no more. It's time to start blaming the real reasons you were fooled and not yourself. Time to start blaming the excessive amounts of unnecessary sugar in the food. Time to start blaming the marketing guys who trick you into buying too much. Time to start blaming the people who make you eat even when you're not hungry. It's time, my friend! Time to take a simple Stepbac® from Overeating and to take back control of your weight and your health. You should never blame yourself or feel bad - or think that you can't fix this yourself. You can!

We know you can start taking a Stepbac® from Overeating, because we know that you already manage your life well in so many other ways. So, of course, you can begin to manage your eating and your weight without manipulation from fake Candyfood and sugar. Think of some of the many tough challenges that you have faced in life over the years. And how you got through them. You have probably accomplished many amazing things, big and small, and you have overcome so many of life's challenges! It might have been in school, at college, at home or at work. Many of our life challenges are much more difficult than learning one small and simple new eating habit. If you can do so many tough and challenging things every day, then of course you can do this - you can easily learn one tiny new habit that will replace all your old overeating habits and help you to control your weight. We know that when you start to take a Stepbac® from all the low-grade food and sugar snacks then you will start to feel energized and confident. You will feel physically and mentally stronger and be able to overcome this challenge without "fake help" from "fake food" promising "fake results" and "fake happiness."

Happiness is all about health, energy and hope, in our opinion. We are sure that you can and will have a better life, a longer life, a healthier life and a happier life if you learn and use the Stepbac® method. Stepbac® will help you experience natural happiness from the joy of things that are possible when you have good health - a bit like when you were a child. You won't be younger in age using Stepbac®, but a healthy body will make you feel younger!

All this new energy will start to appear when you start taking a Stepbac® from Overeating. Your weight gain will stop and if you want to lose weight, then you can control your eating and lose some weight every day until you hit your natural weight. It will take a while, so be patient - remember your energy and confidence will start to go up every day too, and you will start to feel more real and natural happiness and less fake happiness (figure 46).

Figure 46

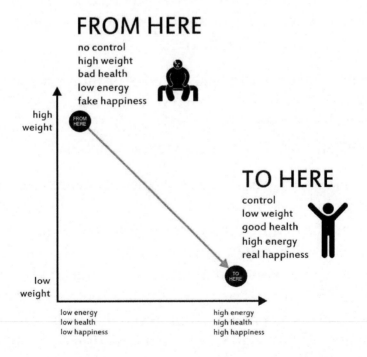

**AFTER using Stepbac®
from Overeating**

FROM HERE

no control
high weight
bad health
low energy
fake happiness

high
weight

TO HERE

control
low weight
good health
high energy
real happiness

low
weight

low energy   high energy
low health   high health
low happiness   high happiness

Another reason that we know you can learn this small and simple Stepbac® from Overeating lifestyle change, is because we did it - and we are as ordinary as sliced bread, especially when it comes to fitness and food.

We are not fitness fanatics, or dieticians or doctors, or psychologists, or cooks, or even foodies. We don't test blenders or mix the best smoothies or climb Everest in Speedos. No way! We are not even members of a gym. We do some watersports and go for some bike rides and walks every week. We are just regular folks. We are probably not much different from you. We are not special. We just felt - like you might be feeling now - that we were getting a little heavier every year from around our mid-thirties, so we had a think about it and over time we came to the conclusion that we were being fooled by the food industry.

Then we started to take - and still take - a Stepbac®. Now we're slim and we control our own weight. That's it. So if we can do it, anyone can do it and you can too! You can learn and use the Stepbac® action.

A very quick recap about things to remember about sugar when you start to Stepbac®. Remember that sugar has no nutritional value. Remember that humans do not need sugar to survive. That if you never ate sugar again, you would not suffer or die from a lack of sugar. Sugar does not give you any benefit - not one. It only steals a benefit from you - it steals your good health (and some of your wealth!). Remember Candyfood is just fake food full of sugar. Fake food promises you a taste of heaven with just one bite, but it's more like a taste of hell. Think too of what we showed you in Chapter 3 about people not eating refined sugar until very recent times - and how sugar is being used by the food industry to trick you into overeating. Remember this: you don't need sugar to be happy. You don't need fake Candyfood to be happy. The very brief feeling of joy that you get after eating a treat or a fake Candyfood snack is a flash of "fake happiness" from the dopamine sugar rush. It didn't change your life for the better. Fake food gives you nothing of value except unwanted calories, extra weight and negative energy. No benefit. No upside. Only the downsides of regret, being overweight and longer-term unhappiness.

Sugar is the drug that is causing you to be overweight. When you quit sugar, you will not want to eat until you're genuinely hungry. And then you will want to eat natural food not Candyfood. It's that simple. When you quit sugar, the cravings leave your body. When you quit sugar you will not want to overeat and you will be back in control of your weight. So do it! Take a simple Stepbac® from Overeating and take back control of your weight and your health. Stop letting your body be a trash can for the food industry. Take a Stepbac® and make your body your most precious possession that will function well, support you and transport you all the way through the rest of your very long, healthy and happy life.

When you start to Stepbac®, remember too that you don't need a sugar hit to fix problems or get through hard times in your life. You will still have problems and challenges in life like we all do. But remember that overeating is a problem not a solution. You don't need to overeat sugary comfort food to fix a problem. Sugar and overeating is a problem! You can't fix a problem with another problem. If you have a problem and you start overeating, then you will have two problems instead of one. To fix problems what you need is happiness, energy and good health, not misery, negative energy and bad health. You can't run fast if you're weighed down by sugar. Sugar only gives you a very short blast of fake happiness and a sugar rush of fake energy, and then it tricks you into overeating and you have to carry the weight and take the blame. Sugar does not give you any real happiness and no real nutritional energy, so it's no help. Time to ditch the Candyfood eating habits. Twice the weight is half the life. It's time to get all your life back.

You will start to feel this new energy as you begin taking a Stepbac® from Overeating. Your weight gain will stop and if you want to lose weight, then you can control your eating and lose a little weight every day until you hit your natural BMI (Body Mass Index, a method used to calculate a person's weight-related health risk) recommended weight. Your energy and confidence will start to go up along the way. That is real and natural happiness, not fake happiness.

You will feel physically and mentally stronger and able to overcome many challenges by yourself and set new goals.

Don't worry about the times that you might have tried to lose weight and failed in the past. Don't worry about not having enough willpower. Forget all that. All the previous attempts that you made at losing weight were probably based on trendy short-term diets or grueling extreme exercise programs. Most of us would fail at those kinds of diets, because they are based on incorrect beliefs about food and weight.

And willpower. You have plenty. Remember you're not alone now. You have Stepbac® on your team! You didn't have a weapon like the Stepbac® method until now. You always had plenty of willpower, but willpower alone can't beat sugar addiction or defend our old prehistoric human brain from modern marketing tricks. Now you have the Stepbac® information with the knowledge about the way sugar hijacks your hunger survival cycle. You have the Stepbac® action to take back control of your natural eating habits and control your weight. You always had the willpower but Stepbac® will supercharge your willpower.

In the beginning you might feel a little self-conscious about using the Stepbac® method, but don't be. Wear the wristband. Take a little step backwards. Just stick with it. Keep doing it. Very soon you will find that it becomes an automatic habit stored and used by your brain. You will very quickly start to take an automatic Stepbac® from tempting but unhealthy food without even thinking about it. You might be surprised that you walk right by chocolate and other candy in the supermarket and think, "Wow, I remember when I used to buy that every day and now I can hardly believe that I just Stepbac® from it without a second thought." You will feel you have the power of Stepbac® in you and you won't be fooled again by fancy wrappers and tempting offers.

What if you're a foodie? Perhaps you're a little worried that food, cooking, eating and sharing food knowledge feels like a big part of your personality? How will your friends react when you start to take a Stepbac®? Perhaps you're the person in your social circles who keeps your friends up-to-date about new recipes, new restaurants and new "blissful" desserts with posts on social media.

Are you thinking perhaps that without food you won't know who you are and have nothing to talk about? Don't worry - you can still be a great foodie and a Stepbaccer too. We can all be foodies, if being a foodie means making and eating delicious healthy food. As a Stepbaccer you will still eat well - but you won't overeat. Remember that you're only taking a Stepbac® from Overeating, not a Stepbac® from "ever eating" nice food again. Stepbac® from Overeating is only a method, and a tool to adjust and manage your eating habits and control your weight. It's not a bread and water life sentence! Quite the opposite. Healthy food is delicious too but in a natural way because natural hunger enhances food flavours and taste. You will discover new and better tastes to replace the Candyfood taste. Candyfood is actually a boring taste because it's always the same... sugary and sweet!

Remember too - do not starve yourself. You are taking a Stepbac® from Overeating - not from eating. Do not under any circumstances ever use "Stepbac® from Overeating" or the Stepbac® method to stop eating for long periods or skipping meals. We repeat: do not under any circumstances ever use "Stepbac® from Overeating" or the Stepbac® method to stop eating for long periods or skipping meals. Stepbac® is a tool to help you control your natural weight. It is not a tool to stop eating and must not be used to stop eating. You must eat a balanced amount of food every day to make sure you get the necessary amount of calories and essential nutrients to be healthy and to stay at your natural weight.

Figure 47

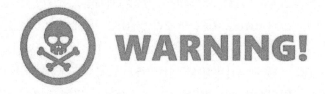

WARNING!

Stepbac® from Overeating

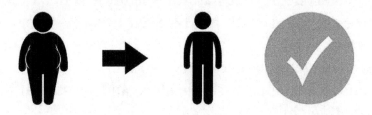

Do NOT stop eating!

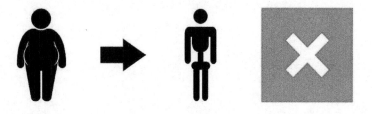

Remember too that we have shown you in this book that overeaters are not happier than natural eaters. We busted the food industry myth that "eating is bliss!" We hope we have busted the myth that you get something special or extra from Candyfood. Remember that eating is no longer "my only friend" or "my only joy in life."

Eating doesn't "make you happier." Are thin people unhappy the whole time because they don't eat? No. Are overweight people happier than thin people? No. These are all part of the myths and marketing fairy tales to trick you into thinking that eating is somehow the gateway to happiness. So don't worry. Your life will not become miserable when you start taking a Stepbac® to eat less. On the contrary. You will be the same person, only much happier and healthier. You will very quickly get used to your new Stepbac® lifestyle and to eating less.

One of the little things we, the authors, started early on to Stepbac® from was putting sugar in our daily coffee. In Spain coffee is delicious and the weather is mild so we often have a coffee outside at a café. In Spain they often serve two quite big packets of sugar with a regular-size coffee. We replaced our habit of adding two sugars with a new Stepbac® habit of just setting the sugar aside. After just a week we put the sugar aside automatically without thinking. And we didn't miss the old sweet taste. We quickly became used to the natural taste of coffee. If we were to add the sugar again now, it would taste much too sweet.

You will find the same thing happening in many other ways. You will enjoy the new taste of food without so much sugar. Your life won't get worse, only better. You will be happier and healthier. The only difference is that when you stop overeating, you will feel much better and have a little more cash in your pocket from not overshopping. That is all. Nothing else will change.

Let's say it again. Nothing else will change. You will be fine without Candyfood and sugar. You will be more than fine. Your life will only change for the better. You will be the same person but feeling better. We know this because it all happened to us.

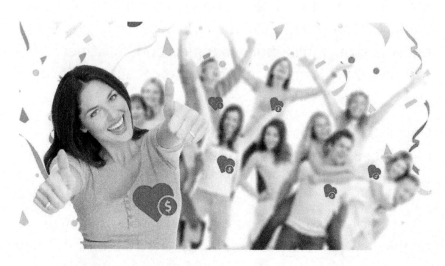

Please donate

Please donate or support us to help others

www.stepbac.com/donate

Congratulations for reading this ebook and well done for learning the Stepbac® method. If this book helped you, then please consider making a donation on our website, big or small, to help us keep Stepbac® books available for everyone free or at the lowest possible price! You can donate using your credit card on PayPal, or on Patreon. You also support us by buying Stepbac® T-shirts and other merchandise.

www.stepbac.com/merchandise

We, the authors Carl and Peter, write and make Stepbac® books available free, or at cost price, to help improve people's health and lifestyle, and to make the world a happier and better place. Our books are completely crowd-funded and we do not receive payments from advertisers or corporate sponsors. A small donation goes towards our daily expenses. Larger donations or recurring monthly donations mean that we can continue to write more books and help more people.

Free Stepbac® ebooks

www.stepbac.com/download

Find free ebooks in the Stepbac® series on www.stepbac.com/download and see how you can download them and share them with friends and family.

Stay in touch

That's all we have for you. Welcome to the Stepbac® movement and look out for new books in the Stepbac® series. You're always welcome to visit us online for more help and inspiration. Thank you sincerely for your support. It means a lot to us and to many people.

www.stepbac.com

Best wishes
Carl and Peter Williams

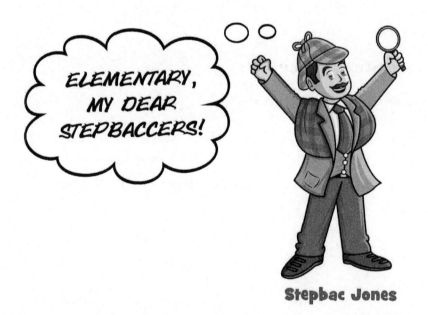

Stepbac Jones

Acknowledgements:

Special thanks to our editor Hannah Pennell for her skill and support.

Also available in the Stepbac® book series:

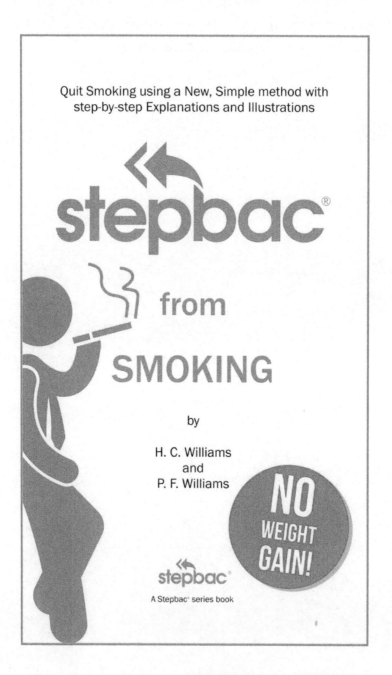

Quit Smoking using a New, Simple method with step-by-step Explanations and Illustrations

stepbac®

from

SMOKING

by

H. C. Williams
and
P. F. Williams

NO WEIGHT GAIN!

stepbac®

A Stepbac® series book

Coming soon in the Stepbac® book series:

Visit www.stepbac.com for more information

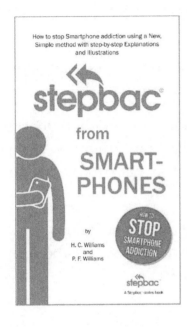

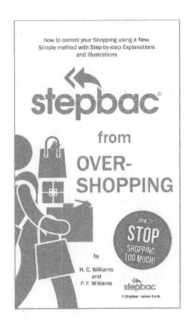

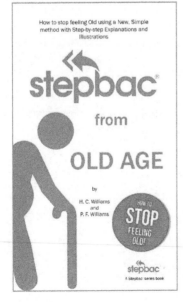

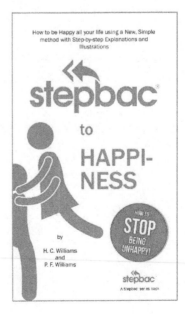

About the authors:

The Stepbac® method was created in 2014 in Barcelona by two tour guides and brothers, Carl & Peter Williams.

They were inspired to write the Stepbac® series of books by a love of nature and their talks with many wonderful tour guests from all over the world.

Carl and Peter developed their own method to stay healthy and happy, which also gave them a strong desire to help others find their way back to the joy and energy of good health.

Carl and Peter are currently writing new books in the Stepbac® series and offer talks and seminars about the Stepbac® method and lifestyle.

Printed in Great Britain
by Amazon

16297191R00122